KU-271-719

Professor Terence Stephenson DM, FRCP, FRCPCH
President, Royal College of Paediatrics and Child Health

SWINE FLU

What Parents Need to Know

Jessica Kingsley Publishers
London and Philadelphia

Disclaimer: Whilst every effort has been made to ensure all medicine doses quoted are correct for the UK at the time of going to press, products can change and countries vary. Always check the label and packaging of any medicine you buy or are prescribed.

The views expressed in this book are the author's personal opinions and are not necessarily the views of other organizations, including the Royal College of Paediatrics and Child Health.

First published in 2009
by Jessica Kingsley Publishers
116 Pentonville Road
London N1 9JB, UK
and
400 Market Street, Suite 400
Philadelphia, PA 19106, USA

www.jkp.com

Copyright © Terence Stephenson 2009

All rights reserved. No part of this publication may be reproduced in any material form (including photocopying or storing it in any medium by electronic means and whether or not transiently or incidentally to some other use of this publication) without the written permission of the copyright owner except in accordance with the provisions of the Copyright, Designs and Patents Act 1988 or under the terms of a licence issued by the Copyright Licensing Agency Ltd, Saffron House, 6–10 Kirby Street, London EC1N 8TS. Applications for the copyright owner's written permission to reproduce any part of this publication should be addressed to the publisher.

Warning: The doing of an unauthorized act in relation to a copyright work may result in both a civil claim for damages and criminal prosecution.

Library of Congress Cataloging in Publication Data
A CIP catalog record for this book is available from the Library of Congress

British Library Cataloguing in Publication Data
A CIP catalogue record for this book is available from the British Library

ISBN 978 1 84905 085 2

Printed and bound in Great Britain by
Athenaeum Press, Gateshead, Tyne and Wear

Contents

AS SAMONaA IN TEGS ie 3 pople ched.

Disclaimer

Whilst every effort has been made to ensure all medicine doses quoted are correct for the UK at the time of going to press, products can change and countries vary. Always check the label and packaging of any medicine you buy or are prescribed.

The views expressed in this book are the author's personal opinions and are not necessarily the views of other organizations, including the Royal College of Paediatrics and Child Health.

Chapter 1

Introduction

It is estimated that up to 30% of children in the world may contract swine flu. Yet a shortage of reliable information about the virus and a bewildering array of media speculation has left many parents anxious and confused. This book presents the key facts about swine flu and explains in plain and simple English what every parent needs to know about the virus, how it may affect their children and the measures to combat it.

Some of the most pressing questions include:

- What is swine flu?
- Just how dangerous is it?
- What are the symptoms?
- What treatments are available?
- Is swine flu more dangerous in children and, if so, why?
- What can we learn from past flu pandemics?

Swine flu is the first major pandemic to sweep across the world since 1968. Inevitably, therefore, much of the evidence I use to draw out answers to these questions is based either on previous flu pandemics over the last century or by extrapolation from seasonal winter flu. Most of the information we have on whether antiviral drugs and flu vaccine benefit children comes from experience with ordinary flu occurring every winter.

This book gives clear guidance on where parents should go for help and advice. It also includes simple tips to help children avoid contracting swine flu and a list of Frequently Asked Questions (Chapter 10) with clear and down-to-earth answers.

If you are confused about swine flu or worried about how best to protect your child over the coming months, read on. For those who want to know the details, I have provided the research evidence where possible to back up the answers. For those of you who want to get straight to the answers, I have provided summary boxes for quick and easy reference.

Sources of information for the public

The views expressed in this book are my personal opinions. They are not necessarily the views of other organizations, including the Royal College of Paediatrics and Child Health.

If you have severe symptoms which are not like flu you should contact your GP or call:

NHS Direct on 0845 4647 (England)

NHS 24 on 08454 24 24 24 (Scotland)

NHS Direct Wales on 0845 4647

I hope this book brings together the essential information you need to know as a parent. Much of it is just common sense and already widely available in many different books, leaflets and websites, but it would obviously take many hours to find it and many more to decipher it. Not an easy thing to do in the middle of the night when you are worried about your ill child. I have tried to pull it together for you, to explain the science behind the swine flu pandemic and to sort the wheat from the chaff.

In the text of this book, I have tried to explain the medical and scientific terms and to avoid jargon. This is one problem with accessing information from the internet, which can often be difficult to understand. Another problem is that although much information is available from the internet, most of it is not filtered for accuracy and some of it is plain wrong. The internet can also be a frustrating tool. Search engines can locate 3,390,000 hits in a tenth of a second, but after trawling the first 20 and still not finding the answer we are looking for, desperation sets in. Should you wish to conduct personal research after you have read this book, I have included a 'Useful Resources' section at the end (see p.154).

LIVERPOOL JOHN MOORES UNIVERSITY
LEARNING SERVICES

Chapter 2

What is swine flu?

Before we look at what swine flu is, we need to talk about what a virus is, then more specifically what an influenza virus is, and then the exciting bit – what swine influenza virus is.

What is a virus?

Human infectious diseases are diseases which can be transmitted or passed on to another human (e.g. chicken pox) or passed from an animal to a human (e.g. rabies from a dog bite or salmonella food poisoning from infected chicken) or from an insect to a human (e.g. malaria, which can be transmitted from a mosquito to a human, but one human can't then infect another directly). There are four types of micro-organisms or bugs that can cause human infections – bacteria, fungi, protozoa and viruses. More recently, a new cause of disease called a prion, which can be transmitted to humans from affected cattle (mad cow disease), has been discovered.

Bacteria

First the bacteria – what most people mean when they refer to 'germs'. Bacteria (singular: bacterium) are a group of single cell micro-organisms, a few thousandths of a millimetre in length. For comparison, the head of a pin is about two millimetres across. Unlike human cells, bacteria have no nucleus (the nucleus is the central core of the cell containing the DNA of our genes). Bacteria exist everywhere, growing in soil, water and in the live bodies of plants and animals.

There are on average 40 million bacteria in a gram of soil and a million bacteria in a millilitre of fresh water. Each person has ten times more bacterial cells in their body than the total number of their own cells, with especially large numbers of bacteria on the skin and in the gut. Bacteria can grow and divide every 20 minutes. One single bacteria cell can give rise to eight million bacteria in 24 hours. The vast majority of the bacteria in the body are harmless and a few are beneficial. However, some bacteria cause infections (such as boils, abscesses, the urinary tract infection cystitis, blood poisoning – also called septicaemia). Many of these bacterial diseases can be passed on to another person (i.e. they are infectious), including whooping cough, tuberculosis, pneumonia and meningitis. The most common fatal bacterial diseases are respiratory infections, with tuberculosis alone killing about two million people a year. Antibiotics are used to treat bacterial infections but antibiotic resistance is becoming common. Most people will have heard of the problems of 'super bugs' (such as MRSA in hospitals) where resistance to antibiotics is an increasing problem.

Fungi

A fungus (plural fungi) is an organism whose cells do contain a nucleus, and fungi are genetically more closely related to animals than to plants. Examples of fungi are as diverse as mushrooms (to eat), yeast (to raise bread and make wine and beer) and bath sponges (to wash our backs)! Most fungi grow as colonies of cells clustered together (as in the examples above) but some species grow as single cells. Fungi are abundant worldwide but individual fungal cells are invisible to the naked eye because of their very small size. They live mainly in soil, on dead matter and on or within plants and animals. Fungi can cause problems in humans, such as candida or yeast infections leading to nappy rash in infants and sexually transmitted infections in adults. These infections can be treated with anti-fungal creams or tablets.

Protozoa

Protozoa (singular protozoon) are single cell micro-organisms also containing a nucleus. Protozoa usually range from ten to fifty thousandths of a millimetre, but can grow up to one millimetre in length and exist in water and soil. Protozoa such as the malaria parasites, trypanosomes (causing sleeping sickness) and leishmania (the flesh-eating bug caught by TV personality Ben Fogle) are causes of parasitic diseases in humans. These parasites can survive outside the human body, allowing their indirect transmission from person to person. An example is giardiasis which can cause abdominal pain and loose stools and be spread between toddlers in nurseries. The most common way that a person can become infected with giardiasis is by drinking water that is contaminated with the giardia intestinal parasite. The giardiasis infection can also be transmitted when an infected person does not wash their hands properly after using the toilet, and handles food that is then eaten by others (the 'faecal–oral route'). Food can also be contaminated if it is washed with infected water.

Other protozoal parasites are transmitted by an insect called a vector. In the case of malaria this is the mosquito; in the case of sleeping sickness, the tsetse fly; in leishmaniasis, the sand fly. Protozoal diseases can be treated with antibiotics.

Viruses

A virus is a tiny infectious agent that can reproduce only inside another host cell. The genes of viruses can be composed of DNA, as are human genes, or of a similar molecule called RNA. DNA stands for DeoxyriboNucleic Acid, the double helix molecule discovered by Watson and Crick in the 1950s, which carries the genetic code of every human being. If the information stored in one person's DNA was printed as a book, the book would be over one billion words long – that's 30,000 times as long as the book you are reading now! RNA is RiboNucleic Acid, a very similar long chain molecule for carrying genetic code in which the deoxyribose sugar in DNA is replaced by ribose. Herpes is a DNA virus. Influenza is an RNA virus.

Viruses infect all types of organisms, including animals, plants and bacteria. Viruses exist everywhere on earth and are the most abundant living thing on the planet. A virus is about one hundredth the size of a bacterium and most cannot be seen even with the strongest light microscope, although they can be demonstrated to exist with a special, more powerful electron microscope. Viruses spread in many ways. Influenza viruses are spread principally by coughing and sneezing, although they can spread by other routes too (see Chapter 8). Rotaviruses are the leading cause of vomiting and diarrhoea in children, causing an estimated half a million deaths worldwide each year. Rotaviruses are transmitted when infected faeces contaminate hands, food, cutlery, dishes, glasses or water and enter the body through the mouth during eating or drinking (again the 'faecal–oral route'). HIV is one of several viruses that are transmitted through sexual contact, through tiny abrasions in the skin which allow the virus to enter the blood stream.

Not all viruses cause disease but many do. The best known example of a viral illness is the common cold. Other viruses such as hepatitis B can cause life-long or chronic infections and the viruses continue to replicate in the body despite the body's defence mechanisms. However, in most cases viral infections in animals cause an immune response that eliminates the infecting virus. These immune responses can also be produced by vaccines that give life-long immunity against a viral infection. **Antibiotics have no effect on**

viruses, but antiviral drugs have been developed to treat both life-threatening and more minor infections.

Prions

A prion is an infectious agent that is composed only of protein and is not living. It is an abnormally-folded form of a protein and causes the brain to degenerate. To date, all prions that have been discovered are transmitted by eating the brain or nerve tissue of an infected animal (e.g. mad cow disease, also known as BSE) or a human brain (cannibalism leading to the disease kuru kuru). BSE stands for bovine (meaning relating to cows) spongiform (causing holes in the brain) encephalopathy (abnormal brain function). In humans the disease is called TSE – transmissible spongiform encephalopathy. All known prion diseases affect the structure of the brain or nerve tissue and all are currently untreatable and are always fatal.

Distinguishing between bacterial and viral infections

The illnesses caused by bacteria and viruses can look very similar. For example, probably only one in ten sore throats is caused by bacteria (usually a circular bug called a strep) and nine out of ten by viruses, but research has shown that it is very difficult to tell one from the other unless a throat swab is taken and examined in the laboratory. It takes a few days to get the swab result, by which time the majority of patients will have recovered irrespective of whether they had a strep throat or a virus. So there is no point in routine swabbing. Faced with a child with a sore throat, there are two equally logical approaches at the first contact with a doctor – treat none with antibiotics or treat all with antibiotics. Since the vast majority of children will recover quickly and fully whether the cause is a bacteria or virus, since all antibiotics can have side-effects and since we want to avoid germs developing resistance, we should use antibiotics as sparingly as possible.

Therefore the best approach is to treat none. Many other viral and bacterial illnesses look very similar. It can often be very hard to distinguish between viral and bacterial pneumonia or viral and bacterial meningitis without further tests.

Influenza

The term *influenza* is derived from Italian and was first used in the Middle Ages when the illness was thought to be due to the unfavorable 'influences' of our stars! You won't find that today in the astrology pages of a newspaper. Changes in medical understanding led to its modification to *influenza del freddo*, meaning 'influence of the cold'.

Influenza, commonly referred to as the flu, is an infectious disease caused by RNA viruses of the orthomyxovirus family. The influenza viruses affect birds and mammals. The most common features of the disease are fever, sore throat, muscle pains, headache, coughing and weakness. Fever and coughs are the most frequent symptoms. In more serious cases, influenza can lead to pneumonia (chest infection) which can be fatal, particularly for the young and the elderly.

Influenza may produce nausea and vomiting, particularly in children, but these symptoms are more common in the unrelated gastroenteritis, which is sometimes confusingly called 'stomach flu'. Gastroenteritis can be due to bacteria (as in salmonella food poisoning) or viruses (most commonly rotavirus – an RNA virus which is the leading cause of diarrhoea among infants and young children).

Typically, influenza is transmitted through the air by coughs or sneezes, creating aerosols containing the virus. Influenza is also transmitted by saliva and nasal secretions. Infection can occur through contact with these body fluids or through contact with contaminated surfaces. As the virus can be inactivated by soap, frequent hand washing reduces the risk of infection.

Influenza spreads around the world in seasonal epidemics, resulting in an estimated 500,000 deaths annually – millions in pandemic years. Three influenza pandemics occurred in the 20th century (1918, 1957 and 1968) and killed tens of millions of people, with each of these pandemics being caused by the appearance of a new strain of the virus in humans. These new strains can appear when an existing flu virus spreads to humans from other animal species, or when an existing human strain picks up new genes from a virus that usually infects birds or pigs. A bird flu strain named H5N1 raised the concern of a new influenza pandemic after it emerged in Asia in the 1990s, but it has not changed into a form that spreads easily between people – yet.

Influenza virus A

There are three types of influenza virus – A, B and C. The type A viruses are the most important for humans and cause the most severe disease. Wild birds and humans are the main reservoirs of influenza A infection. If a new strain of virus arises, it can cause devastating outbreaks in domestic poultry or give rise to human influenza pandemics.

The disease is transmitted by:

• direct contact

• droplet infection (through coughing or sneezing)

• contact with non-living objects which have been freshly soiled with discharges from the nose or throat of an infected person, such as a drinking glass used by an infected person.

An infected person can pass the disease to someone else for at least five days after the onset of the disease, and up to ten days in the case of an infected child. Occasional cases originate in humans transmitted from animals, e.g. pigs or chickens.

Effects of influenza viruses

Influenza virus infection kills the tiny cells in the lining of the airways. This starts in the nose (rhinitis), then spreads down the throat (pharyngitis) and windpipe (tracheitis) and, in the most severe cases, to the airways of the lungs (bronchitis and bronchiolitis). The lining of the airways consists of 'hair cells', tiny cilia which beat back and forward, sweeping dust, bugs and other debris up from the lungs and airways as mucus, keeping them clean. If this 'muco-ciliary escalator' is damaged, mucus and secretions collect in our airways and we sniffle, cough and sneeze in an effort to eject the fluid. Also, whenever cells die, inflammation results. The airway lining becomes thickened, red and sore.

In the most severe cases, this inflammation extends all the way down in the lungs, beyond the small airways and into the lung tissue itself – viral pneumonia. Pneumonia literally means lung infection, commonly called a chest infection. This can interfere with the ability of the lungs to get oxygen into the body and provides the perfect environment for bacteria to creep in as uninvited guests. The normal defences of the lining of the airways and lungs are weakened by the effects of the flu virus and a secondary bacterial pneumonia can result. The commonest germs are called *streptococcus pneumonia* (pneumococcus), *staphylococcus aureus* (some of which are MRSA) and *klebsiella pneumonia*.

The naming of influenza viruses

Each wave of influenza A virus is given a particular code. Examples in humans include:

- H1N1 which caused Spanish flu in 1918, and the 2009 flu pandemic
- H2N2 which caused Asian flu in 1957
- H3N2 which caused Hong Kong flu in 1968
- H5N1 avian flu, a recent pandemic threat.

The letters 'H' and 'N' in these abbreviations refer to two proteins on the surface of the flu virus – haemagglutinin and neuraminidase. Influenza viruses are made up of a central core of RNA genes with a covering coat. From this outer envelope, spikes containing hemagglutinin (H) proteins stick out and between these spikes sit the mushroom-shaped neuraminidase proteins.

A haemagglutinin is a substance that causes red blood cells in a test-tube to agglutinate or stick together. Examples of haemagglutinins include antibodies (see Chapter 7) and the proteins that determine whether we have an A, B or O blood group. However, bacteria, viruses and parasites can be the source of blood agglutinins as well. In terms of influenza virus, the role of the haemagglutinin molecule is to anchor the virus to any human cell the virus tries to enter. The H protein is used to prepare anti-flu vaccines because the H protein molecule is what the human immune system uses to recognize the virus as foreign (see Chapter 7).

Neuraminidase (N) is a protein that helps flu viruses to eat their way through mucus secretions. The antiviral drugs oseltamivir (Tamiflu®) and zanamivir (Relenza®) work by blocking the N protein.

Many subtypes of influenza virus are endemic in humans, dogs, horses and pigs and hence we hear of bird flu, human flu, swine flu, horse flu and dog flu. In pigs, horses and dogs, influenza symptoms are similar to humans, with coughing, fever and loss of appetite.

How come humans get swine flu and bird flu but not dog flu?

Suppose a cell is simultaneously invaded by strains of influenza virus that normally infects different species (e.g. birds and humans). These flu viruses can exchange genes. In 1957 and 1968 the influenza types responsible for those outbreaks are thought to have arisen through the exchange of genes between avian and human viruses. Genes code for proteins and proteins are made up of chains of building blocks called amino acids. The new virus can still infect humans because some of its genetic code is from the human strain. But humans have no defences against the new virus because our immune system does not 'remember' ever seeing the amino acid segments coded for by the genes from the bird strain of influenza (see Chapter 7 on immune defences). This kind of genetic exchange does not seem to occur with dog or horse flu strains.

Also, influenza infections can happen directly from animals to humans too but they are rarely passed on to other human beings so a pandemic does not take hold. For example, the H5N1 avian influenza has infected human beings many times in the past ten years but has not led to subsequent infections, human to human. Because successful crossovers are rare, there is little research in humans that we can rely on now. Hence, much of the advice with regard to swine flu is extrapolated from what we know about regular winter flu. Only a few crossovers, mostly from swine, have ever led to widespread infection in humans (e.g. in 1918). In 2009, it seems to have happened again. H1N1, the current variant, is thought to be the descendant of two unrelated swine viruses, one of them a derivative of the 1918 human virus.

Swine flu

Swine influenza (also called hog flu or pig flu) is an infection by any one of several types of swine influenza virus. Swine influenza virus is any strain of the influenza family of viruses that is endemic in pigs. Influenza type A virus outbreaks in pigs are the most common but rarely cause death. In pigs, swine influenza produces fever, lethargy, sneezing, coughing, difficulty breathing and decreased appetite. Direct transmission of an influenza virus from pigs to humans is occasionally possible (this is called zoonotic swine flu). In all, about 50 human cases are known to have occurred since identification of influenza subtypes became possible in the mid-20th century. These have resulted in six deaths. Symptoms of zoonotic swine flu in humans are similar to those of seasonal influenza – fever, sore throat, muscle pains, headache and coughing.

Cooked pork products are safe to eat as the virus cannot be transmitted by eating foods. Cooking kills the virus. People with regular exposure to pigs are at increased risk of swine flu infection but these strains of swine flu rarely pass from human to human.

When swine flu does catch hold in human populations, as during a pandemic, human-to-human transmission of swine flu spreads in the same way as seasonal flu – through coughing and sneezing. In April 2009 a novel flu strain appeared that apparently combined genes from human, pig and bird flu viruses. Initially called 'swine flu', this virus emerged in Mexico before spreading to the US and then around the world. The virus is named swine flu because its surface proteins are most similar to flu viruses that usually infect pigs and these have been spreading in North American pigs for years. The new virus is genetically related to recent swine influenza viruses but has a genetic make-up or 'finger print' not previously detected among viruses infecting either swine or human populations. There is no evidence that the infection first started in Mexico after transmission from a pig to a human. This particular H1N1 virus is spreading between people and we don't know whether it will infect pigs.

The World Health Organization (WHO) officially declared the outbreak to be a 'pandemic' on 11 June 2009. This virus is an H1N1 variant but so was the 2008 seasonal variant. So why is this one affecting more people and why does last year's anti-flu vaccine not protect against the 2009 pandemic?

Because, although they are both H1N1 types, the H1 protein in the 2009 version is sufficiently different from the H1 in the 2008 version that the new version can spread quickly because people have no natural defences against it.

Pandemic declared

The outbreak began in Mexico in March 2009. Although the Mexican government closed many of Mexico City's public facilities to try to contain the spread, and some countries hastily cancelled flights from Mexico, by early June the virus had spread globally and the WHO declared the outbreak to be a pandemic. The WHO declared a Pandemic Alert Level of six (out of a maximum six) describing the degree to which the virus had been able to spread among humans. The pandemic level describes spread of the virus rather than its severity. On a separate scale for severity, WHO assessed the global severity as moderate. Raising the alert to level six led countries to consider shutting borders, banning events and curtailing travel. In addition, at phase six, many pharmaceutical companies switched from making winter flu vaccine to pandemic-specific vaccine, potentially creating shortages of immunization to counter the normal winter flu season.

Why were there so many deaths in Mexico while infections in other countries appeared to be relatively milder? It may be that Mexico had many more cases than were officially recognized – a 'silent epidemic'. As a result, perhaps Mexico was reporting only the most serious cases which would give a skewed initial estimate of the case fatality rate.

An early study from the US published in May 2009 found that 94% of patients with confirmed swine flu infection had a fever and 92% had a cough. The virus has continued to spread worldwide, especially in the Southern Hemisphere which was in its winter flu season. In previous pandemics, it has taken six months for influenza viruses to spread as far afield as the new

The WHO Pandemic Alert Levels

Phase	Description
Phase 1	No animal influenza virus circulating among animals have been reported to cause infection in humans.
Phase 2	An animal influenza virus circulating in domesticated or wild animals is known to have caused infection in humans and is therefore considered a specific potential pandemic threat.
Phase 3	An animal or human–animal influenza reassortant virus has caused sporadic cases or small clusters of disease in people, but has not resulted in human-to-human transmission sufficient to sustain community-level outbreaks.
Phase 4	Human-to-human transmission of an animal or human–animal influenza reassortant virus able to sustain community-level outbreaks has been verified.
Phase 5	The same identified virus has caused sustained community-level outbreaks in two or more countries in one WHO region.
Phase 6	In addition to the criteria defined in Phase 5, the same virus has caused sustained community-level outbreaks in at least one other country in another WHO region.
Post peak period	Levels of pandemic influenza in most countries with adequate surveillance have dropped below peak levels.
Post pandemic period	Levels of influenza activity have returned to the levels seen for seasonal influenza in most countries with adequate surveillance.

swine flu virus did in six weeks but international travel and trade is much more common now.

Is it safe to travel?

A number of countries, especially in Asia, initially enforced strict quarantines of airline passengers showing flu symptoms, including passengers seated near to any infected persons. A number of airlines also began pre-screening passengers before they travelled.

WHO is not recommending travel restrictions related to the outbreak of the swine flu H1N1 virus. Limiting travel and imposing travel restrictions would have very little effect on stopping the virus from spreading and would be highly disruptive to the global economy. Swine flu H1N1 has already been confirmed in many parts of the world. Nor does the WHO think that entry and exit screenings in each country would work to reduce the spread of this disease.

Initial fears allayed

The most notorious flu pandemic is thought to have killed at least 50 million people worldwide in 1918–19. However, evidence mounted throughout May 2009 that the symptoms of the current swine flu pandemic were milder than health officials initially feared. Most of the first 342 confirmed cases in New York City were mild. Similarly, Japan reported 1048 mostly mild flu cases and no deaths, with the government re-opening schools stating that the virus should be considered more like a seasonal flu. By August 2009, with the Southern Hemisphere winter finishing, Australia had almost 28,000 confirmed cases out of a population of 21 million. Of course the number of unconfirmed cases was much higher. However, there were only around 100 deaths attributed to swine flu in the first three months that the pandemic hit Australia and just over 3000 people admitted to hospital. This compares to the 1500–3000 deaths which are put down to seasonal flu each year in Australia and the 15,000 deaths in the 1918–19 pandemic of Spanish flu when the population of Australia was only six million.

Chapter 3

What is a pandemic and what can we learn from previous pandemics?

In June 1914 Gavrilo Princip, a Serbian nationalist, fired a shot which echoed around Europe. The assassination of Archduke Franz Ferdinand heralded the start of World War I in which 662,000 healthy, young British soldiers died. On 1 July 1916 my grandfather fought at the Battle of the Somme in which 19,500 men were killed on the first day. He survived the war only to face an even greater threat on demobilization.

The year 1918 saw the onset of the Spanish flu A (H1N1) pandemic which claimed the lives of up to 50 million people around the world. Like World War I, it particularly killed previously healthy, young adults. My grandfather also survived that scourge. Perhaps his rural life as a farmer in north-west Ireland saved him. Influenza, like other viruses infecting the lining of the lungs and airways, is easily spread by coughs and sneezes which propel fine droplets containing the virus through the air. He was protected by the 'inverse square' principle – the further you are away from something, the less it is likely to affect you. Examples include the law of gravity, 'personal' music players and X-rays – that's why your dentist pops out of the room when taking an X-ray of your teeth. The isolated existence on my grandfather's farm made the chances of him meeting an infectious person much lower than in a densely populated city.

It is estimated that between 20% and 40% of the world's population were affected by Spanish influenza, which emerged in 1918 in Europe and then travelled to the US, Africa and Asia. Between 20 and 50 million people were killed, including millions of young adults – more people died as a result of the disease than in World War I; 250,000 people died in Britain alone. The attack rate and mortality of the disease were highest among those aged between 20 and 50. The illness characteristically took hold very quickly, with patients who began feeling unwell in the morning sometimes dead by night time. This is not the case with the 2009 swine flu. Many patients who lived through the first few days of the Spanish flu were killed by complications such as pneumonia. A virus with the severity of Spanish flu has not been seen since, possibly because of the advancements in medical care, living conditions and nutrition during the 20th century.

What is a pandemic?

The word pandemic comes from the Greek 'pan', all, and 'demos', meaning people. A human pandemic is an epidemic of infectious disease spreading across a large region, for example a continent, or even worldwide. A widespread disease that is stable in terms of how many people become sick from it from year to year is not a pandemic. In this case the disease is said to be *endemic*. The biggest killer each year in the world is pneumonia, causing four million deaths per year worldwide. Forty million people live with HIV and there are three million deaths per year from AIDS. Each year around the globe, ten million children die before the age of five years. That's one every three seconds. Most die from endemic diseases. For example, malaria is endemic in many parts of the world, killing one African child every 30 seconds, but it is not a pandemic. Throughout history there have been a number of pandemics of bacterial infections, such as the Black Death and tuberculosis, and of viral infections, such as smallpox. A more recent example of a viral pandemic is HIV. Routine seasonal flu, occurring every winter in both hemispheres, is excluded from the definition of a pandemic but causes epidemics.

Pandemics are characterized by the number of people affected but also in many pandemics apparently young and healthy people tend to be affected as severely as elderly people and more vulnerable groups. When a pandemic does emerge, it may occur in more than one wave, several months apart. In the 2009 swine flu outbreak, the UK government repeatedly warned about the likelihood of a second wave of swine flu some time after the initial outbreak, possibly as much as nine months later.

How do pandemics arise?

As influenza is caused by a variety of strains of the flu virus, in any given year some strains can die out while others create epidemics, while yet another strain can cause a pandemic. Typically, in the two flu seasons each year (one per hemisphere), there are between three and five million cases of severe illness and up to 500,000 deaths worldwide. Although the incidence of influenza can vary widely between years, approximately 36,000 deaths and more than 200,000 hospitalizations are directly associated with influenza every year in the US. Even during a winter where the incidence of flu is low, up to 4000 deaths may be attributed to flu in the UK. This can rise much higher in epidemic years. For example there were an estimated 13,000 deaths in winter 1993–94 which were due to flu and 29,000 deaths in 1989–90.

New influenza viruses are constantly evolving genetically, creating a multitude of strains until one appears that can infect people who are immune to the existing strains. This new variant then replaces the older strains as it rapidly sweeps through the human population, often causing an epidemic. However, since the new strain will still be reasonably similar to the older strains, some people will still have some immunity to it. However, about three times per century, the influenza virus develops such different forms of the two surface proteins that a pandemic occurs because there is no overlap with existing immunity in the population. Everybody is susceptible and the novel influenza virus will spread uncontrollably, leading to a pandemic.

Previous flu pandemics (and false alarms)
1918 Spanish flu (H1N1)
The most famous and lethal outbreak was the 1918 flu pandemic which lasted from 1918–19. It is not known exactly how many died, but estimates range from 20–100 million people worldwide, with the World Health Organization settling on 45–50 million. Between September 1918 and April 1919, approximately 675,000 deaths from the flu occurred in the US alone. The majority of deaths were from bacterial pneumonia, a secondary bacterial infection as a consequence of serious viral influenza.

The 1918 flu pandemic was truly global and the unusually severe disease killed probably somewhere between 2% and 20% of those infected, as opposed to the more usual flu epidemic mortality rate of 0.1%. Another unusual feature of this pandemic was that it mostly killed young adults, with 99% of pandemic influenza deaths occurring in people under 65, and more than half in young adults between 20 and 40 years old. This is unusual since influenza is usually most deadly to the very young (under age 2) and the very old (over age 70).

Swine influenza was first proposed to be a disease related to human influenza during the 1918 flu pandemic. But current thinking is that in 1918 the virus moved from humans to pigs and not vice-versa. In the spring of 1918, influenza in humans spread rapidly all over the world and became prevalent throughout China. In October 1918, a disease diagnosed as influenza appeared in Russian and Chinese pigs. Similarly, in the late summer or early autumn of 1918, a disease not previously recognized in swine, and closely resembling influenza in humans, appeared in pigs in the American Mid-West. The evidence, albeit fragmentary from 90 years ago, points to the spread of virus from humans to swine. The virus was recovered from pigs more than a decade later in the first isolation of influenza virus from a mammalian species.

The current H1N1 form of swine flu appears to be one of the descendants of the strain that caused the 1918 flu pandemic. As well as persisting in pigs, the descendants of the 1918 virus have also circulated in humans through the 20th century, contributing to seasonal epidemics of H1N1 influenza.

1957 Asian flu (H2N2)

The Asian influenza epidemic was first identified in the Far East in February 1957. Due to advances in scientific technology, the virus was quickly typed and by August 1957, limited supplies of a vaccine were available. It took just three or four months for the virus to spread from Southeast Asia to Europe and North America, and by autumn 1957 every part of the world had experienced cases.

The disease struck in two waves, in the autumn of 1957 and then in early 1958, with very high rates of illness and an increase in fatalities. This is an example of the potential 'second wave' of infections that can develop during a pandemic. Elderly people proved most vulnerable, although infection rates were highest among school children, young adults and pregnant women. Although the Asian flu pandemic was not as severe as the Spanish flu, about two million people died worldwide, including 70,000 people in the US and 30,000 in the UK.

1968 Hong Kong flu (H3N2)

The 1968 pandemic was milder than that of 1957 and spread more slowly than previous pandemics, affecting mostly the very old and those with underlying medical conditions. Symptoms were relatively mild and the death rate was not as high as in previous epidemics. The number of deaths between September 1968 and March 1969 for this pandemic was 33,800 in the US, making it the mildest pandemic in the 20th century. About one million people are estimated to have died worldwide.

It is possible that the 1968 pandemic may have been milder than the previous two because those exposed to the 1957 strain may have built up a partial protection against the virus. Also, in later pandemics antibiotics were available to control secondary infections and this may have helped reduce mortality compared to the Spanish flu of 1918. Breathing machines and oxygen supplies were not available in 1918. Alternatively, the decrease in severity may be because the flu virus is evolving in favour of better infectivity but less virulence. A virus that kills its host or sends them to bed will be transmitted less.

There is another piece of good news in terms of the 2009 swine flu outbreak. A small viral protein, PB1-F2, seems to be one marker of how severe the disease will be in humans. It was present in the strains responsible for the 1918, 1957, and 1968 pandemics but the 2009 version of H1N1 does not carry it.

1976 Fort Dix USA (H1N1)

An army recruit at Fort Dix died and four other soldiers were later hospitalized. The cause of death was a new strain of swine flu, a variant of H1N1. It was detected only from 19 January to 9 February and did not spread beyond Fort Dix. Forty-three million Americans were later vaccinated (see Chapter 7). It is difficult to say why the outbreak at Fort Dix petered out, although it had the potential to be fatal, and yet the outbreak in Mexico City became global; the difference was not due to a vaccine since the outbreak ceased within weeks, long before the vaccine was available.

1977 Russian flu (H1N1)

This outbreak was unusual in being very age-restricted, affecting mostly young adults and children. Russian flu, red influenza or red flu first came to attention in November 1977 in the former Soviet Union. It quickly became apparent that this rapidly spreading epidemic was almost entirely restricted to persons less than 25 years of age and that, in general, the disease was mild. The younger age distribution of affected people was put down to the absence of H1N1 viruses in humans after 1957, and the dominance of the H2N2 strain in 1957 and the H3N2 strain in 1968. The theory was that H1N1 had been circulating in a milder form as seasonal flu between 1918 and the 1950s and that in 1977, everyone over the age of 25 had some immunity to this variant of H1N1. The degree of change in the 2009 form of H1N1 compared to the virus circulating previously must be significantly greater since all ages seem vulnerable this time round.

1988 Zoonosis Wisconsin USA (H1N1)

In 1988, swine flu virus killed one woman and infected others. The woman became ill after visiting the hog barn at a county fair. An H1N1 strain of swine influenza virus was identified.

Influenza-like illness was widespread among the pigs exhibited at the fair, and three quarters of the swine exhibitors tested positive for swine flu infection but no serious illnesses

LIVERPOOL JOHN MOORES UNIVERSITY
LEARNING SERVICES

were detected among this group. A small number of health care personnel who had contact with the patient developed mild influenza-like illnesses with laboratory evidence of swine flu infection. However, there was no wider outbreak.

Direct transmission of a swine flu virus from pigs to humans is occasionally possible (called zoonotic swine flu). In all, 50 cases are known to have occurred which have resulted in a total of six deaths. The 2009 H1N1 virus is not zoonotic swine flu, as it is not transmitted from pigs to humans, but from person to person.

Doctor speak

epizootic = an epidemic in a non-human species

panzootic = a disease affecting animals of many species, especially over a wide area

zoonosis = a disease passing from animals to humans

1997 Bird flu (H5N1)

Flu in birds is mostly a mild disease. However, some flu strains cause more extreme disease and significant mortality, producing sudden severe illness and almost 100% mortality within a few days. As the virus spreads rapidly in the crowded conditions seen in the battery farming of chickens and turkeys, these outbreaks can cause huge losses to poultry farmers.

A strain of influenza virus called H5N1 causing 'avian influenza' or simply 'bird flu' is endemic in many bird populations, especially in Southeast Asia. Avian flu does not normally infect species other than birds or pigs but the first documented infection of people with the H5N1 virus occurred in Hong Kong in 1997, causing severe lung disease in 18 people, six of whom died. The disease emerged again in February 2003 and again in December 2003. Since 2003, this virus has caused the largest and most severe outbreaks in poultry on record. In December 2003, infections in people exposed to sick birds were identified in four Asian countries (Cambodia, Indonesia, Thailand and Vietnam) and more than half of these people died. Most cases occurred in previously healthy children and young adults. By 2008, according to the WHO, 385 people around the world had been infected with H5N1 and 243 of them had died.

At present, H5N1 is mainly an avian disease and there is little evidence suggesting efficient human-to-human transmission. So far person-to-person spread, if it has occurred, has done so with difficulty. In almost all cases, those infected have had extensive physical contact with infected birds. However, due to the high lethality and virulence of H5N1 and its endemic presence, the H5N1 virus was the world's pandemic threat in the 2006–07 flu season. Much of our preparedness for swine flu is because countries have been gearing up for a potential H5N1 influenza pandemic since then.

Known flu pandemics

Name of pandemic	Date	Deaths	Subtype involved
Spanish flu	1918–1920	20–100 million	H1N1
Asian flu	1957–1958	1–2 million	H2N2
Hong Kong flu	1968–1969	0.75–1 million	H3N2

Do flu pandemics particularly affect children and young people?

In community studies of seasonal flu, school-aged children have had the highest rates of influenza infection. Influenza illness demonstrates annual attack rates of between 15% and 42% in preschool- and school-aged children in the US. A similar pattern was seen during pandemics in the last century and is already apparent early in the current swine flu pandemic (see Figure 1).

In addition, during winter flu, young children also seem to be at higher risk of hospitalization for influenza infection than are healthy adults over the age of 50. Finally, children younger than 24 months of age are consistently at higher risk of hospitalization than are older children, and the risk of hospitalization is highest in the youngest children. Of 182 patients hospitalized at Montreal Children's Hospital with laboratory-proven influenza between 1999 and 2002, 34% were younger than 6 months of age.

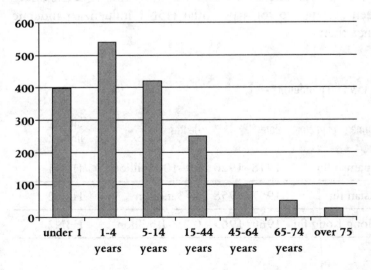

Figure 1. Age distribution of consultation rates for flu-like illness in the UK. Consultation rates are per 100,000 of the population per week.

Was SARS a flu pandemic?

No. SARS (Severe Acute Respiratory Syndrome) is due to a different virus called a coronavirus. SARS was another potential pandemic, like avian flu, which did not take off. There was one near pandemic of SARS, between November 2002 and July 2003, with 8096 known infected cases and 774 deaths worldwide. Within a matter of weeks in early 2003, SARS spread from Southern China to infect individuals in 37 countries around the world. As of May 2006, the spread of SARS has been fully contained.

Chapter 4

What are the symptoms of swine flu?

Illnesses are made up of symptoms and signs. A symptom is what a patient feels and describes to their doctor. A sign is something the doctor detects when examining you. So if you have appendicitis, you might describe the symptom of tummy pain but the doctor would elicit the sign of tenderness when pressing on your belly.

The symptoms of swine flu are much the same as those of ordinary winter flu. Symptoms of swine flu can start suddenly one to two days after infection.

Typical symptoms of swine flu

- Fever (a high body temperature of over 37°C or 98.6°F).
- Feeling cold or hot.
- Cough.
- Runny nose.
- Sore throat.
- Sneezing.
- Reddened mouth, throat and nose.
- Fatigue or tiredness.
- Headache.

- Aching joints and muscles.
- Irritated, watering or red eyes.
- Loss of appetite.
- Stomach upset, feeling sick or vomiting.
- Abdominal pain.
- Diarrhoea.

Some sufferers will have all or most of these symptoms whereas others will have a milder form of the disease with fewer symptoms. You do not have to suffer a 'full house' to be diagnosed with swine flu (see Diagnosis below).

Upper respiratory tract infection

Because the commonest features of flu affect the nose, throat and upper airways, it is one cause of a clutch of childhood illnesses known as upper respiratory tract infections (URTIs). URTI is a catch-all term used when we are not sure which exact bug is causing this common cluster of childhood symptoms. The common cold is the most common URTI but other viral causes are influenza and parainfluenza viruses (which can cause croup in toddlers). Whooping cough, on the other hand, is an example of a bacterial URTI.

Diarrhoea

Diarrhoea is not commonly a symptom of influenza in adults, although it has been seen in some human cases of the H5N1 'bird flu'. The 2009 swine flu outbreak has shown an increased percentage of patients reporting diarrhoea and vomiting. In children, gastro-intestinal symptoms such as vomiting, diarrhoea and abdominal pain tend to be more of a feature than in adults.

Influenza in young infants

In babies, the features of flu are much more non-specific. There may be brief episodes when breathing stops or there may be lethargy, irritability and poor feeding.

Signs of swine flu

- Reddened mouth, throat and nose.

- Raised temperature (a high body temperature of over 37°C or 98.6°F and may reach 39–40°C).

- There may be a fleeting red rash, which can be mistaken for measles.

- In uncomplicated cases, when a doctor listens to the chest with a stethoscope there is little abnormal to hear. If there is pneumonia, the doctor may hear abnormal breathing sounds through the stethoscope.

Measuring fever in children

- Do not routinely measure temperature by the oral or rectal routes.

- Do not use forehead chemical thermometers.

- Ideally use an electronic thermometer in the armpit. Failing that, an old-fashioned mercury in glass thermometer will do.

Progress of the illness

The incubation period (time from viral infection to onset of illness) of influenza is short and ranges from one to three days. What might a parent expect to see day by day? The progression of a viral illness can vary greatly between one child and another.

- At first, the child may be non-specifically unwell, perhaps feeling cold and tired and not sure why. An infant may be 'grizzly' and more difficult to settle.

- High fever usually follows fairly soon after the onset of symptoms, and indeed sometimes is the very first sign of illness.

- This is often accompanied by the other features of aching, sore throat, coughing, runny nose and sneezing. A child may be laid low by these symptoms for a few days and take to their bed. Other children have milder symptoms and are still up and about although they feel 'rough' and perhaps just want to watch TV and not be disturbed.

- The worst of the symptoms of aching and fever usually subside after 48–72 hours but coughing, runny nose and sneezing may persist for a week.

- If a child develops diarrhoea and vomiting, this will usually coincide with the peak of the illness. However, in babies and toddlers, loose stools can persist for several weeks after the child has otherwise recovered. This is because in a minority of children, a 'secondary' intolerance to the special lactose sugar in milk results from the viral infection of the lining of the gut.

- Abdominal pain ('gastric flu') can be a prominent symptom.

The average length of illness in untreated children with a confirmed case of normal seasonal flu is about five days (longer in children under two years – six days; shorter in children over five years – four days). Research has shown that by day five of the illness, however, only a third of children will have returned to school or normal activity. Furthermore, in one in ten children, symptoms of influenza persist for more than two weeks. In swine flu, the average length of illness is four days but this can range anywhere from two to eleven days in different children with more mild or severe disease.

Most children who have contracted swine flu recover within a week and do not suffer complications, even without being given antiviral medication.

Diagnosing swine flu

It can be difficult to distinguish between the common cold and influenza in the early stages of these infections, but in flu there is usually a higher fever with a sudden onset and extreme fatigue. Many people are so ill that they are confined to bed for several days, with aches and pains throughout their bodies which are worse in their backs and legs.

The symptoms most reliably seen in influenza are:

Symptom	Rate in patients with influenza
Fever	70–85%
Cough	85–95%
Runny nose	70–90%

Since anti-viral drugs are effective in treating influenza only if given early (see Chapter 6), it is important to identify cases early. During a swine flu outbreak, doctors will consider swine influenza infection as a possibility in all patients with sudden onset of fever and respiratory symptoms. Of the symptoms listed above, the combinations of fever with cough, sore throat and/or nasal congestion are enough to make the diagnosis sufficiently likely to offer treatment. Data from the US suggests that during a swine flu outbreak in summer, when other viral respiratory tract infections are rare, clinical suspicion is usually correct and thus patients with any of these combinations of symptoms may be offered anti-viral drugs without testing.

Misdiagnosis of swine flu

In winter, distinguishing swine flu from other common winter viral illnesses may be more difficult. For example, every winter there is an epidemic in young children of bronchiloitis (meaning the small airways of the lungs – the bronchioles – become inflamed). This is due to a virus known as RSV (Respiratory Syncytial Virus) and leads to hundreds of children, especially infants less than one year, being admitted to hospital, usually peaking between November and February. Children with RSV have fever, cough, runny nose and increased rate of breathing – all very like swine flu. Once in hospital, there is a rapid, same-day test available to confirm the presence of RSV in a swab taken from the back of the nose.

However, most milder cases and older children will remain at home where this test is not feasible. Tamiflu® is not a treatment for RSV but nor will it make RSV worse. The problem here is that children could be given Tamiflu unnecessarily for no benefit, decreasing stockpiles of the drug and exposing children to unnecessary side-effects.

An alternative, and potentially more serious scenario is where a child with flu-like symptoms is diagnosed clinically with swine flu (either face to face or by telephone), given Tamiflu and remains at home but is actually in the early stages of a more serious disease. For example, I have heard of a new case of diabetes (which presented with the non-specific symptoms of headache and abdominal pain) and a case of teenage meningitis (fever and headache) being treated initially with Tamiflu. Given how non-specific the symptoms of swine flu are, especially in the early phase of the illness, this is almost inevitable, especially when there are very large numbers of cases. The only advice I can give is to ask parents to remain vigilant and keep an open mind even when the label of 'swine flu' has already been applied. If the child deteriorates markedly or the features change, parents should seek further advice. Paediatricians are taught, 'Listen to the parent, he or she is telling you the diagnosis.' Parents know their children well and many will have seen viral illnesses and URTIs in their children before. Your concerns are important.

Emergency situations

There are some emergency situations when you should always seek immediate medical attention. If your child has any of the following symptoms, seek medical advice:

- Your child is unresponsive, unconscious, floppy, limp, or impossible or difficult to wake.

- Your child has a new breathing problem that is so severe that they are unable to finish a sentence.

- Your child feels that their throat is closing off and they are unable to swallow saliva or drooling excessively.

- Your child shows a change in colour – blue or greyness – particularly around the lips or mouth.

- Your child is having their first ever fit (also called a seizure or convulsion).

To help parents, I have suggested below some more detailed warning signs for all children under 16 years old. The majority of children are expected to be managed in the community. However, breathing failure, overwhelming diarrhoea and vomiting, shock and encephalitis (brain inflammation) can occur in children suffering from swine flu.

Equally well, the features in the list below may be due to another severe illness or due to both swine flu and another illness (e.g. meningitis) occurring in the child at the same time.

Children with the following should be referred to the nearest general hospital emergency department:

- **Severe breathing distress**: lower rib cage indrawing, indrawing of the breast bone, grunting or noisy breathing when calm.

- **Increased breathing rate**: measured over at least 30 seconds. More than 50 breaths per minute if under one year, or more than 40 breaths per minute if over one year.

- **Child looks grey or blue**.

- **Breathing stops intermittently**: more than 20 second pause in breathing (many normal children have shorter pauses or sighs in their breathing, especially when asleep).

- **Evidence of severe dehydration or shock**: not drinking, sunken eyes or fontanelle (the soft spot at the top of the forehead of a baby under 12 months. A tense or bulging fontanelle is a sign of meningitis as is sudden onset of squint in an ill child).

- **Altered conscious level**: strikingly agitated or irritable, seizures, or floppy infant.

- **Causing other clinical concern**: e.g. a rapidly progressive or an unusually prolonged illness.

If your child is completely unable to move their chin down to touch their chest, this can be a sign of meningitis. Immediately seek medical attention.

Not drinking is an important warning sign in young children because they can become dehydrated quickly (see Chapter 5 on treatment of swine flu symptoms for details of how much fluid to give your child). In contrast to fluids, we do not really worry about a child who is not eating. Once over the age of a year, most children have enough calories stored in their body to cope with not eating for several days during an acute illness. The exception is young babies – see the box below.

Babies – feeding during illness

Young babies who are still breast or bottle fed, especially under four months, cannot tolerate as long an interval between feeds as older children who can fast safely overnight and miss meals. For babies, their diet is entirely liquid and their reserves of body fat are less. If not drinking, then they are not eating either and there is an increased risk of low blood sugar causing drowsiness. They are then even less likely to wake and be alert for the next feed.

Assessment of children less than one year old

Clinical signs can be non-specific in the very young. I would emphasize that all infants less than one year old should be examined by a doctor or a delegated health care professional with appropriate training and experience before issue of Tamiflu. This is in accordance with UK Department of Health guidance and has been agreed by the British Medical Association and Royal College of General Practitioners.

Rashes and flu

Influenza does not commonly cause a rash but can do so. The rash is red, flits about the body and is not so specific as to aid in diagnosis. In children, the illness can also be associated with a 'heat rash' because of the raised temperature. This is a fine, pink rash, sometimes slightly raised, which tends to wax and wane as the child's temperature fluctuates. A rash can also occur as a side-effect of most drugs (Tamiflu, antibiotics, ibuprofen) – either looking similar to a heat rash or consisting of raised wheals and itchy blotches like hives or nettle stings. These pink rashes blanch when pressure is applied. So use the 'tumbler test' to demonstrate that when you press firmly with the base of a glass tumbler on an affected area of skin, the pink colour of the spots turns to normal skin colour.

Non-blanching rashes should never be ignored

If your child has a non-blanching rash, i.e. it remains visible using the tumbler test, this should never be attributed to flu. This may be a marker of a serious infection, although fortunately this is not usually the case. If there are large, flat, purple skin patches, some of which may look like a fresh bruise, and these do not blanch on the tumbler test, these are called purpura. A purpuric rash is due to blood seeping from the tiny blood vessels into the skin tissues and is often a feature of blood poisoning or meningitis due to bacteria called meningococcus. This is a very serious disease and you need to get your child medical attention as soon as possible. If there is no fever, the purpura may be due to a blood clotting disorder, but let the doctors sort that out. Purpura hardly ever occurs in viral infections (there are always exceptions – it can do so in rare cases of severe chicken pox).

If the non-blanching rash is made up of multiple, pin-head sized pink or purple spots in the skin, these are called petechiae. A petechial rash is also due to blood leaking from the tiny capillary blood vessels into the skin, either due to infection or the build up of pressure in the blood vessels. So a petechial rash can also signal meningococcal infection but, unlike purpura, we sometimes see petechiae in other bacterial and viral infections. If the petechiae are confined to the neck, face, eyelids and scalp, this is usually a result of something causing increased pressure in the veins of the neck. For example, choking, retching, vomiting, prolonged coughing or screaming. Of course, there may still be a serious underlying infection causing these symptoms. Increase in pressure is also why facial petechiae occur when someone is throttled around the neck or a victim of hanging. Finally, petechiae confined to one cheek or earlobe are usually the result of the pressure from a slap mark. In this situation, there will be no fever.

Laboratory diagnosis of swine flu

Because the symptoms are not specific to swine flu, a definite diagnosis of confirmed swine flu requires laboratory testing of a respiratory sample (a simple nose or throat swab). But, as growing the swine flu virus in the laboratory takes too long, other techniques to detect swine flu are available. A nasopharyngeal aspirate (a sample of mucus obtained from the back of the nose using a special type of swab) can give a result the same day using a lab technique called immunofluorescence. Essentially, the lab has a stock of antibodies which recognize the protein coat of the virus and stick to it. The antibodies are tagged with a fluorescent dye which lights up bright green under the microscope. Hence the presence of the virus can be detected although the viruses themselves are much too small to see even with a microscope.

If other body samples are obtained in which there are fewer virus particles, such as a throat swab or spinal fluid from a suspected case of meningitis, then a different technique called PCR can be used. This stands for Polymerase Chain Reaction and is used to detect the genes of the swine flu virus. Scientists take a DNA copy of the swine flu virus RNA which makes up the genetic code of influenza viruses. They then amplify the tiny amounts of the DNA molecule until they reach detectable levels. Although the technique itself can take as little as 30 minutes to perform, these tests are usually run in batches, sometimes only in certain centres, and therefore the results can take much longer to return.

Why does my child describe feeling cold when they are hot to touch?

Fever is common early in swine flu, with body temperature rising from a norm of around 36.7°C to 38–39°C (approximately 100–103°F). Exceptionally, the temperature may reach 40°C. As a result, often the first symptoms are chills or a chilly sensation. This is because the viral infection resets your body's thermostat – your body is fooled into thinking it needs to be hotter than the normal 37.6°C. You feel cold and your muscles start to shiver to generate heat. You climb into bed under a duvet with a hot water bottle and a hot drink in an effort to warm up. Eventually your body temperature rises to the new set-point, let's say 39°C. You now have a raised temperature but the chilly symptoms cease.

Why does my child sweat when their temperature is falling?

As your body resets its thermostat back down to, say, 38°C, either through medication or by naturally fighting the fever, your symptoms change to those of fever. You feel hot (because your body temperature of 39°C is now above the new set-point of 38°C) and you start to sweat to try to lose heat. You kick off the duvet, open the windows and switch on the fan until your temperature falls to 38°C when you feel better again.

Lightwood's Law

A useful way of thinking about bacterial and viral infections is 'Lightwood's Law' — bacteria focus and viruses spread. Examples of bacterial infections are a boil on the neck, a tooth abscess, pneumonia affecting one lobe of one lung. The body's defences tend to stop the bacteria spreading more widely (except in very serious and overwhelming infections like blood poisoning) and pus forms locally. However, viruses spread very quickly throughout the body even in a patient with perfectly normal defences. This viraemia (the spread of viruses via the bloodstream) explains why we have so many different symptoms in flu and why we have so many aches and pains. The virus gets into the lining of the upper airway, mouth and nose causing a sore throat and runny nose, coughing and sneezing; into the muscles causing pain in the back and legs (myalgia); into the membranes around the brain (causing neck stiffness, pain at the backs of the eyes and discomfort from bright lights); into the lining of the gut causing vomiting and diarrhoea. We appear flushed (because a high temperature causes the blood vessels in the skin to open up in an effort to lose heat) or pale (because until our temperature rises, the blood vessels in the skin close up in an effort to conserve heat). In severe influenza, a patient may also look pale because of shock (the blood pressure is low or the heart is not pumping well) or blue (so called cyanosis when the lungs are not getting enough oxygen into the bloodstream).

Chapter 5

Treatment of swine flu symptoms

The symptoms which can be treated at home with common remedies are pain, fever and dehydration. There are also measures parents of young babies can take to reduce the chance of the fever from swine flu increasing the risk of cot death. These are each dealt with in the sections which follow – first pain control, then temperature control, then giving fluids.

General advice to parents and carers

Parents and carers should:

- be aware of the antipyretic (combating fever) interventions available (see below)
- offer their child regular fluids (see below – if breastfeeding then continue as normal)
- look for signs of dehydration:
  - sunken fontanelle
  - dry mouth
  - sunken eyes
  - absence of tears
  - poor overall appearance

- encourage their child to drink more fluids and consider seeking further advice if they see signs of dehydration
- know how to identify a non-blanching rash (see Chapter 4)
- check their child during the night
- keep their child away from nursery/school while the fever persists and notify the nursery/school of the illness.

Parents and carers of a child with swine flu should seek further advice if:

- the child has a fit
- the child develops a non-blanching rash (see Chapter 4)
- they feel that the child's health is getting worse
- they are more worried than when they last received advice
- the fever lasts longer than seven days
- they are distressed or concerned that they are unable to look after their child.

Pain

Swine flu can cause localized pain, such as headache or sore throat, or a more generalized feeling of aching all over due to involvement of muscles and joints. In either case, there are two types of medicine widely available for home use for the relief of pain in children (see below). It used to be a common presumption that young children feel less pain and have less need for painkillers (analgesics). There is no scientific basis for this – it is simply that young children find it more difficult to express themselves and we, as parents, find it more difficult to distinguish the cry of pain from the cry for a feed or a nappy change.

Successful management of pain depends on identifying its source and assessing what, if anything, eases or aggravates it. It is important to consider not only the pain itself but also the psychological aspects (e.g. fear, especially during a pandemic with huge media scares) and the child's surrounding environment (see below for distraction techniques). Relief of pain therefore requires more than just giving painkilling drugs.

In children, the relief of fear and anxiety is particularly important. Careful explanation in terms that the child can understand (what might happen, what it might feel like and what will be done to reduce the pain) can help the child to cope. A reassuring environment, the presence of a parent and the comfort of a special teddy or a favourite DVD will often add to the relief achievable with painkilling drugs.

Parents can help a great deal. You will know how your child normally copes with pain and what usually brings relief. You can help interpret symptoms by knowing if your child is naturally quiet and shy or noisy and extroverted.

Assessment depends heavily on the age and development of the child and on his or her capacity to communicate. In very young children, crying, irritability, grimacing and loss of interest in play or eating can be clues to pain in children too young to describe their experience or who are suffering in silence.

Assessing your child's pain

Children over four years old are usually more able to report pain and its intensity can be assessed using graded pictures of facial expression (Figure 2), diagrams (Figure 3 – which

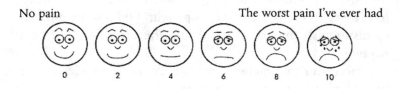

No pain   The worst pain I've ever had

Figure 2. A simple 0–10 pain scale which young children can use.

can be in colour – red for the most severe pain and blue for no pain) or visual analogue scales (Likert scales – Figure 4). A simple six-face scale of pain self-reported by the child (Figure 2) can be used to monitor the effectiveness of pain relief in children.

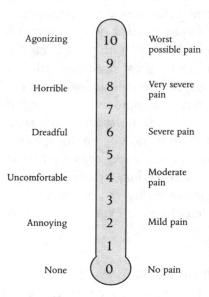

Figure 3. 'Thermometer' pain scale for older children.

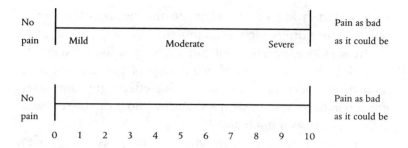

Figure 4. The Likert scale for children's pain assessment – an older child simply marks an X at the point on the line which they feel corresponds to their current level of pain.

Both drug and non-drug approaches to pain relief should be considered. Their use in a complementary way can enhance pain relief.

Non-drug approaches

Rocking, cuddling and 'rubbing it better' often help children in pain. Most non-drug approaches build on the principle of 'distraction therapy'. Familiar activities such as play, reading stories, listening to music or watching a DVD, chosen by and suited to the child, can be structured to interest him or her and keep their mind off the pain they are suffering. All can be effective additions to drug treatment but carers need to remember that some compliant children may co-operate adeptly while in fact suffering in silence.

Medicines for pain relief – paracetamol and ibuprofen

Adequate and regular dosing is crucial. 'As required' dosing of medicines is best avoided: controlling renewed pain when painkillers wear off is harder than maintaining a stable level of pain control.

Paracetamol has painkilling and anti-fever (see below) properties but does not lessen inflammation. Paracetamol has very few side-effects in normal doses given regularly over a week and is less of an irritant to the stomach than anti-inflammatory drugs such as ibuprofen.

In overdose, paracetamol can cause fatal liver disease. If your child has an accidental overdosage of paracetamol seek immediate emergency treatment – side-effects are sometimes not apparent for four to six days. The overdose can be reversed if the child is seen immediately.

Anti-inflammatory painkillers such as ibuprofen (sometimes referred by the abbreviation NSAIDs – non-steroid anti-inflammatory drugs) are particularly useful for the treatment of children with pain and inflammation.

As aspirin may cause a rare but fatal condition called Reye's syndrome in children with a fever, aspirin should be avoided for children under 16 years.

The same two classes of drugs (paracetamol and ibuprofen) can be used to help keep a child's temperature down. The doses in both situations are the same and are given after the next section on fever control.

Fever
Keeping a child's temperature down
Some drugs can reduce body temperature – these are called antipyretics. The UK National Institute of Clinical Excellence offers the following advice:

- Consider either paracetamol or ibuprofen as an option if the child appears distressed or is unwell.

- Do not routinely give anti-fever drugs to a child with fever with the sole aim of reducing body temperature.

- Do not administer paracetamol and ibuprofen at the same time but consider using the alternative anti-fever drug if the child does not respond to the first drug.

- Do not use anti-fever drugs with the sole aim of preventing febrile convulsions.

- Do not rely on a change in temperature one to two hours after administration of anti-fever drugs to differentiate between serious and non-serious illness.

- Tepid sponging is not recommended (it is effective at lowering body temperature but only whilst you continue to sponge – the temperature rebounds up again shortly after you stop).

- Do not over or under dress a child with fever.

The child under one year with a fever – risk of cot death

A cot death (also called SIDS – Sudden Infant Death Syndrome) occurs when a previously well infant is put to sleep and then found dead for no apparent reason some hours later. Children aged less than one year are at risk of cot death – the rate is about one per thousand infants. The highest risk is at three to four months. Factors which appear to increase the risk include:

- winter time
- infant sleeps on his or her front (also called prone sleeping)
- parents are smokers
- younger mothers
- over-heating – either through too many bed clothes or the bedroom being too warm
- bottle fed baby rather than breast fed
- poorer families
- children born close together
- child shares a bed with an adult who smokes or has drunk excessive alcohol.

If an infant has a fever, their risk of over-heating is greater.
Advice to reduce the risk is:

- put the baby to sleep on his or her back ('the back
  to sleep' campaign)
- tuck the bedding in firmly at the bottom, avoid
  duvets and pillows, place the feet of the infant at the
  foot of the cot ('the feet to foot' campaign)
- keep the room temperature no higher than 16–18°C
- use a number of separate blankets rather than a thick
  quilt so that you can vary the amount of covering
  depending on how hot it is in the room and how
  hot the baby is
- never cover the baby's head
- never sleep on a sofa with a baby.

The catch is that in winter, well-meaning parents hear from
the weather forecast that it is going to be a cold night and
turn up the central heating and swaddle their baby more. The
danger is that the child will over-heat, especially if they have
a fever with swine flu.

Medicines to reduce fever

Medicines can be used to treat pain and fever. They work
best if given at regular intervals throughout the day in the
recommended doses, rather than waiting until the child
complains of fever or discomfort and then giving a single
dose. It would not be harmful to give both paracetamol and
ibuprofen to your child (they do not 'interact' with one
another) but this is not recommended as there is no evidence
that this improves temperature control. Therefore, do not
give paracetamol and ibuprofen at the same time but consider
substituting the alternative anti-fever drug if the child does
not respond to the first drug you try.

Giving medicines to children

Medicines vary in form and are administered in different ways.

Young children and infants who cannot understand will usually take medicine from someone they know and trust – a parent or main carer. It is important that those who give medicines know about the medicine and how to give it. Occasionally a medicine has to be disguised. On rare occasions a child may have to be restrained for the medicine to be administered. Then, especially, the child should be comforted and reassured.

- *Under 2 years*. Administration by parents if possible.

- *Two- to five-year-olds* need a calm, gentle, firm and efficient approach after they have been told what is happening. Never ask a toddler, 'Can I give you your medicine?' They are likely to say, 'No.' Play and acting out may help them understand. Rewards and an acceptable drink as a 'chaser' encourage further collaboration.

- *Five- to twelve-year-olds* also need encouragement, respect for their trust, and an explanation attuned to their understanding.

- *Over 12 years*. At this age children must have a proper understanding of what is happening and share in the decision making as well as the responsibility. They must feel in control.

Forms of medicine
Liquids

Children under five years are unlikely to accept tablets if offered, though they may well swallow whatever they find in a cupboard, or indeed in any other place. Keep all medicines out of the reach of young children, ideally in a locked cabinet.

Older children also often prefer liquids. Liquid formulations sometimes have the disadvantage of an unpleasant taste and the accuracy of the dose may be less. Sugar-free medicines should be used whenever possible. The taste of medicines may be disguised by flavouring or by mixing them with favourite foods or drinks. Do NOT mix medicines in a baby's bottle.

Domestic teaspoons vary in size and are not a reliable measure. Five millilitre plastic syringes to give liquids into the mouth are a welcome development. They are available from pharmacists.

Tablets

Tablets are convenient, compact and stable. For the medicines mentioned in this book, the tablets can be crushed and the capsules emptied into food to make them acceptable to the child. Always check with your pharmacist about other medicines – some special medicines (for example for epilepsy and cystic fibrosis) work only if swallowed intact.

Down a feeding tube

If your child has an illness requiring a plastic feeding tube (down the nose or directly through the abdominal skin into the stomach), liquid medicines can be given via the tube, provided that the liquid formulation flows easily down the tube and does not block it. The medicine should be 'washed' through with warm water. If medicines are given to a newborn infant via a nasogastric tube, then sterile water must be used.

If your child has an illness which requires continuous feeding down the tube, feeding should be discontinued for 15 minutes before giving a medicine down the tube.

The licensing of medicines

Before a pharmaceutical company can promote a drug, it must obtain a licence. The company must demonstrate the safety, quality and effectiveness of the drug when given in the dose and for the disease and age group recommended. In the UK, doctors can legally prescribe drugs without a licence. Prescribing may be unlicensed (e.g. as a different formulation) or outside the terms of the licence (so-called off-label prescribing, e.g. in a different dose, or for a different disease or age group. Prescribing outside the licence is relatively common for hospitalized children. In an average neonatal intensive care unit, 90% of infants receive unlicensed or off-label drugs. In general practice, between 10% and 30% of prescriptions for children are unlicensed or off-label drugs.

Just because a medicine is not licensed for children it does not mean it is unsafe. Some medicines have been around for so long that no one would benefit from seeking a licence. The situation is that:

- those who prescribe for a child should choose the medicine which offers the best prospect of benefit for that child, even if it is unlicensed

- it will be obvious from the figures quoted above that the informed use of some unlicensed medicines or licensed medicines for unlicensed applications is necessary in paediatric practice

- in general, it is not necessary to take additional steps, beyond those taken when prescribing licensed medicines, to obtain the consent of parents, carers and child patients to prescribe or administer unlicensed medicines or licensed medicines for unlicensed applications.

Aspirin

Aspirin must be avoided in all children under 16 years because of the risk of a potentially fatal complication called Reye's Syndrome. Young children with a fever are most at risk.

Paracetamol

Paracetamol (often referred to as Calpol® although this is just one trade name) is available over the counter in supermarkets and pharmacies without a prescription.

Side-effects

Side-effects are rare but rashes and, much more rarely, blood disorders have been reported. The best known side-effect is liver damage, which can be fatal, following deliberate or accidental overdose.

Licensed use

Not licensed for use in children under 2 months by mouth.

Indications and dose

When to take: for aches, pains or fever with discomfort.

How to take: by mouth. (Paracetamol suppositories are also available to be given by rectum if your child has intractable vomiting — seek the advice of your pharmacist.)

Dosage: Note the doses in the table opposite are in milligrams (mg) of paracetamol not millilitres (ml). For children, paracetamol in liquid form is usually dispensed as 125 mg in each 5 ml (see 'Paracetamol formulations' below) but a stronger adult liquid is available — be careful.

Paracetamol dose for fever after the flu vaccine in young infants

If high fever (over 38.5°C) develops after childhood immunization, your infant can be given a dose of paracetamol and, if necessary, a second dose six hours later. (Ibuprofen may be used if paracetamol is unsuitable — see below.) Seek medical advice if the fever persists.

For post-immunization fever in an infant aged two to three months, the dose of paracetamol is 60 mg. (The dose

Paracetamol doses

Age	Dose	Frequency
2–3 months	30–60 mg	every 8 hours as necessary
3–12 months	60–120 mg	every 4–6 hours (maximum 4 doses in 24 hours)
1–5 years	120–250 mg	every 4–6 hours (maximum 4 doses in 24 hours)
6–12 years	250–500 mg	every 4–6 hours (maximum four doses in 24 hours)
12–18 years	500 mg	every 4–6 hours; *for severe symptoms* 1 gram (1000 mg, i.e. two 500 mg tablets) every 4–6 hours (maximum four doses in 24 hours)

of ibuprofen is 50 mg on a doctor's advice.) An oral syringe can be obtained from any pharmacy to give the small volume required.

Paracetamol formulations

Paracetamol comes in a variety of tablets and liquids (called formulations) with numerous different brand names such as Calpol, Panadol®, etc.

- *Tablets and caplets*: paracetamol 500 mg.
- *Capsules*: paracetamol 500 mg.
- *Soluble tablets (dispersible tablets)*: paracetamol 500 mg.
- *Paediatric soluble tablets (paediatric dispersible tablets)*: paracetamol 120 mg.
- *Oral suspension 120 mg/5 ml (paediatric mixture)*: paracetamol 120 mg/5ml. Sugar-free versions

can be ordered by specifying 'sugar-free' on the
prescription. Brands include Calpol Paediatric,
Calpol Paediatric sugar-free, Disprol® Paediatric,
Medinol® Paediatric sugar-free, Paldesic®, Panadol
sugar-free.

- *Oral suspension 250 mg/5 ml (mixture)*: paracetamol
  250 mg/5 ml. Brands include Calpol 6 Plus,
  Medinol Over 6, Paldesic.

- *Suppositories*: paracetamol 60 mg.

How should I give paracetamol?

- *Tablets* should be swallowed with a glass of water or
  juice. Your child should not chew the tablets.

- *Dispersible tablets*. Dissolve the tablet in a glass of
  water or squash. Your child should drink it straight
  away. Make sure that they drink it all. You can also
  give the mixture to your child using a spoon or oral
  syringe.

- *Liquid medicine or syrup*. Measure out the right amount
  using a medicine spoon or oral syringe. You can get
  these from your pharmacist. Do not use a kitchen
  teaspoon as it will not give the right amount.

- *Suppositories*

  ○ Wash your hands with soap and hot water.

  ○ Unwrap the suppository.

  ○ Your child should be lying on his or her side or
    front.

  ○ Hold one buttock gently to one side so that you
    can see the back passage.

  ○ Hold the suppository with the rounded end
    close to the back passage.

- Use one finger to push the suppository gently into the back passage. It needs to go in by about 2 cm.

- Your child should stay lying down for about 15 minutes so that the suppository doesn't come out.

- Wash your hands again with soap and hot water.

Note: If your child empties their bowels (does a poo) within 30 minutes of inserting a suppository, you will need to insert another one.

Ibuprofen

Ibuprofen (often referred to as Brufen® or Junifen® although these are trade names) is available over the counter in supermarkets and pharmacies without a prescription. It is one of a family of drugs called non-steroidal anti-inflammatory drugs (NSAIDs).

Side-effects

In regular full dosage ibuprofen combines anti-inflammatory, painkilling and anti-fever properties. It has fewer side-effects than other NSAIDs.

Gastro-intestinal side-effects

Gastro-intestinal side-effects (discomfort, nausea, diarrhoea, and occasionally bleeding and ulceration) have been reported with all NSAIDs. Ibuprofen is associated with the lowest risk in this family of drugs. Children appear to tolerate NSAIDs better than adults and gastro-intestinal side-effects are rare in those taking ibuprofen for short periods.

Asthma

All NSAIDs have the potential to worsen asthma although in my experience this is very rare in practice.

Cautions

Ibuprofen should be used with caution in children with previous allergy to any NSAID — which includes those in whom attacks of asthma, facial swelling or a rash like nettle stings have been caused by any NSAID. Ibuprofen should be used with caution in children with kidney, heart or liver problems or active or previous gastro-intestinal ulceration or bleeding. Consult your child's doctor before giving this over-the-counter remedy.

Licensed use

Not licensed for use in children under three months or with a body weight under five kilograms.

Indications and dose

When to take: for mild to moderate pain, inflammation or fever with discomfort.

How to take: by mouth.

Dosage: Note the doses in the table opposite are in milligrams (mg) of ibuprofen not millilitres (ml). For children, ibuprofen in liquid form is usually dispensed as 100 mg in each 5 ml.

IBUPROFEN DOSE FOR FEVER FOLLOWING FLU VACCINE IN YOUNG INFANTS

For infants aged two to three months the dose of ibuprofen is 50 mg (on a doctor's advice) as a single dose, which can be repeated once after six hours if necessary. An oral syringe can be obtained from any pharmacy to give the small volume required.

Ibuprofen formulations

Ibuprofen comes in a variety of tablets and liquids (called formulations) with numerous different brand names such as Junifen, etc.

Ibuprofen doses

Age	Dose	Frequency
Child 3–6 months	50 mg	3 times daily; maximum 30 mg/kg daily in 3–4 divided doses
Child 6 months–1 year	50 mg	3–4 times daily; maximum 30 mg/kg daily in 3–4 divided doses
Child 1–4 years	100 mg	3 times daily; maximum 30 mg/kg daily in 3–4 divided doses
Child 4–7 years	150 mg	3 times daily; maximum 30 mg/kg daily in 3–4 divided doses
Child 7–10 years	200 mg	3 times daily; maximum 30 mg/kg (maximum 2.4 grams = 2400 mg) daily in 3–4 divided doses
Child 10–12 years	300 mg	3 times daily; maximum 30 mg/kg (maximum 2.4 g) daily in 3–4 divided doses
Child 12–18 years	300–400 mg	3–4 times daily; (maximum 2.4 grams = 2400 mg) daily in 3–4 divided doses

- *Tablets*: coated, ibuprofen 200 mg. Brands include Arthrofen®, Ebufac®, Rimafen®.

- *Oral suspension*: ibuprofen 100 mg/5 ml. Ibruprofen tablets and ibruprofen oral suspension sugar-free may also be prescribed by a doctor. Brands include Calprofen®, Fenpaed®, Feverfen®, Nurofen® for Children, Orbifen® for Children.

Dehydration
How much fluid should my child drink?

Not drinking is an important warning sign in young children because they can become dehydrated quickly. A child weighing ten kilograms (22 pounds) needs a litre (1000 millilitres or 1.75 pints) of fluid in every 24-hour period. For children weighing less than ten kilograms (22 pounds), the calculation is 100 millilitres (just under four fluid ounces) in every 24 hours for every kilogram (2.2 pounds) of body weight. So a six-month-old baby weighing six kilograms would need 600 millilitres (20 fluid ounces) in every 24 hours.

Young babies who are breast or bottle fed may take, on average, even more fluid in each 24-hour period. Usually around 150 millilitres (one quarter of a pint or five fluid ounces) for every kilogram (2.2 pounds) of body weight in every 24 hours.

Older children need less fluid per kilogram. They still need 100 millilitres per kilogram for the first ten kilograms of body weight. But for the next ten kilograms they need only 50 millilitres per kilogram and thereafter only 20 millilitres per kilogram. So a child weighing 25 kilograms (about four stone) needs in every 24 hours:

$$10 \times 100 \text{ ml} = 1000 \text{ ml for the first 10 kilograms of body weight}$$

$+$ $\quad$ $10 \times 50 \text{ ml} =$ another 500 ml for the next 10 kilograms of body weight

$+$ $\quad$ $5 \times 20 \text{ ml} =$ another 100 ml for the last 5 kilograms of body weight

$=$ $\quad$ **1600 ml of fluid in total**

These are all basic minimum figures in well children. A child who is ill and losing extra fluid through sweating, vomiting or diarrhoea will need larger amounts. Since drinking liquids may make the child feel sick, the secret is 'little and often'. A teaspoonful is five millilitres. Aiming to give a one-year-old weighing ten kilograms a minimum of 1000 millilitres in each 24 hours is 40 millilitres per hour or two teaspoonfuls every 15 minutes. This is more likely to stay down than offering a large volume in a bottle every hour. The thirsty child may gulp this down and equally rapidly vomit it back up. Remember, if the child is asleep for 12 out of every 24 hours, and therefore not drinking during these periods, then in this example you would need to get four teaspoonfuls into the child every 15 minutes during the waking periods.

Oral rehydration soltuions for children with diarrhoea or vomiting, such as Dioralyte® and Electrolade®, are available from all pharmacies. These accelerate the correction of rehydration and replace essential salts as well as providing calories.

Summary box – Treatment of swine flu symptoms

- Children with swine flu should:
  - get plenty of rest
  - drink plenty of liquids
  - if necessary, take paracetamol or ibuprofen to relieve the fever and muscle aches associated with the flu
  - avoid taking aspirin because this can lead to Reye's syndrome, a rare but potentially fatal disease of the liver
  - teenagers should avoid alcohol and cigarettes.

Since swine flu is caused by a virus, antibiotics have no effect unless prescribed for secondary infections such as bacterial pneumonia (chest infection) – see Chapter 6.

Antiviral medication like Tamiflu can help (see the Chapter 6).

However, the majority of children infected with the virus make a full recovery without requiring medical attention or antiviral drugs.

Antiviral drugs and the role of antibiotics

Antivirals against influenza

There are two classes of antiviral drugs which have been used against influenza viruses. These are neuraminidase blockers and M2 protein blockers. Neuraminidase blockers are being used against swine flu virus infections since swine flu is resistant to the M2 blockers. Neuraminidase is an enzyme that helps invading viruses to eat their way through mucus secretions in the nose and airways as they approach a human cell. The letter 'N' in H1N1 stands for neuraminidase.

Neuraminidase blockers

- Antiviral drugs such as oseltamivir (trade name Tamiflu®) and zanamivir (trade name Relenza®) are neuraminidase blockers that are designed to halt the spread of the virus in the body.

- Tamiflu and Relenza are both medicines of the same type but Relenza comes as an inhaler and is recommended for use in pregnancy, whereas Tamiflu comes as a capsule or liquid. Both drugs reduce symptoms and some complications of swine flu.

Different strains of influenza viruses have differing degrees of resistance against these antivirals. Genetic changes known to make the flu virus resistant to Tamiflu or Relenza have been looked for and not found in 2009 swine flu. Although currently there is no evidence that swine flu is resistant to Tamiflu, it is impossible to predict what degree of resistance might develop during a pandemic.

M2 blockers

Swine flu in the 2009 outbreak has been found to be resistant to amantadine and rimantadine. This high level of resistance may be due to the easy availability of these M2 blockers as part of over-the-counter 'cold' remedies in some countries and their use to prevent outbreaks of influenza in farmed poultry. They are therefore not recommended in the current swine flu outbreak.

Use of antivirals against swine flu

The antiviral medications Tamiflu and Relenza are available throughout the UK to treat people with swine flu. Antivirals are not a cure for swine flu but can make the illness milder and make the patient feel better more quickly because they:

- reduce the length of time a person is ill by around one day
- relieve some of the symptoms
- reduce the potential for serious complications such as pneumonia.

The World Health Organization (WHO) rated the UK as one of the best-prepared countries for a swine flu pandemic. The UK has large stocks of Tamiflu and Relenza — at the end of summer 2009 there are enough to treat half the population. New orders of Tamiflu have been placed to increase UK supplies to 50 million courses, enough to treat 80% of the population. Currently, antiviral drugs are being given to all those diagnosed with swine flu as a precautionary measure.

Antiviral drugs work best if the course is started soon after getting sick (within 2 days of symptoms). Successful treatment with Tamiflu in children requires starting treatment as soon as possible, when influenza virus replication in the respiratory tract is maximal. In a study of children aged 14 years and under who attended UK general practices during a winter influenza season and received a clinical diagnosis of influenza infection, 64% presented within two days of becoming ill. So if the same is true during a pandemic, about two thirds of children will be able to start Tamiflu within this critical first two days of the illness. Commencement of therapy is not generally recommended outside this period, although it may be considered for critically ill, hospitalized patients.

Key message

Tamiflu works best if given within 48 hours of the start of the swine flu illness.

How do we know antivirals work for children with flu?

Three research trials involving 1500 children with clinical influenza were conducted prior to 2005, of whom 977 children had laboratory-confirmed winter influenza. The children were less than 12 years of age. A clinical diagnosis of influenza was made if the temperature was above 37.8°C and the child had at least two of the following symptoms:

- cough
- headache
- muscle aches
- sore throat

- fatigue

and no clinical evidence of a bacterial infection. The diagnosis was made by a healthcare professional in a community in which there was an influenza outbreak. In two thirds of these children there was also laboratory confirmation of influenza.

In all three trials, the antiviral drug (Tamiflu in two and Relenza in the other) was compared to a placebo (dummy drug). Children were randomly allocated (effectively by toss of a coin) the active antiviral drug or the dummy, which looked identical. We can place more faith in such well designed, randomized comparisons with placebo (see the Cochrane Review below).

Tamiflu reduced the average duration of illness by 26% (36 hours) in healthy children with laboratory-confirmed influenza. The reduction was only 7.7% (10 hours) in 'at risk' (asthmatic) children. Relenza reduced the median duration of illness by 24% (1.25 days) in healthy children with laboratory-confirmed influenza. No data in 'at risk' children are available for Relenza. Tamiflu also prevented complications of influenza, in particular, ear infections. Although there was a trend towards a reduction in complications with inhaled Relenza, the evidence was not absolutely water-tight.

One of the problems is that many of the children included in these studies did not have laboratory proof of infection with influenza virus. If the child did not have influenza, then he or she could not benefit from anti-influenza drugs. This tends to dilute the apparent benefit in these research studies. Similarly, in the UK over three winter seasons of flu, influenza virus was detected in less than half of swabs submitted in children attending UK general practices with influenza-like illness. In pandemic influenza, however, a greater proportion of children presenting with influenza-like symptoms are likely to have true influenza. The real size of the benefit of antiviral drugs may therefore be greater in a pandemic situation.

What are the side-effects of Tamiflu?

The most common side-effect of Tamiflu in adults is nausea, which occurs twice as frequently as with a placebo (the dummy tablet used to compare with Tamiflu). In trials of this medicine, approximately 10% of patients reported nausea (feeling sick) without vomiting, and an additional 10% experienced vomiting. Insomnia has also been reported.

In children younger than 16 years there have been a number of reports (mainly from Japan) of neuropsychiatric events (such as delirium, hallucinations, confusion, abnormal behaviour leading to injury, convulsions and encephalitis). Many believe that the increased reports of neuropsychiatric events in Japanese children are due to an increased awareness of influenza-associated side-effects, increased access to Tamiflu in that population and intensive monitoring of adverse events. However, a study funded by the company Roche (who make Tamiflu) noted a higher rate of mood disorders among young people aged 17 years or less receiving Tamiflu compared to those who received no antiviral treatment.

Research on antiviral drug side-effects from the early summer 2009 UK swine flu outbreak

During April and May 2009, a number of London schools were advised to close due to confirmed cases of swine flu in schoolchildren and Tamiflu was offered to close contacts in the schools. These close contacts were offered Tamiflu as a prophylactic precaution after a classmate received a diagnosis of swine flu. Prophylaxis means using a medicine as a prevention in well children who have been in contact with a case but are themselves not yet showing any signs of illness, rather than as a treatment for children who are already ill. This is sometimes called post-exposure prophylaxis.

The importance of this piece of research is that the scientists deliberately excluded any of the contact children who developed flu-like symptoms. In studies of Tamiflu side-effects in patients who have flu, part of the problem is deciding whether the 'adverse events' reported by the patients are true side-effects of the drug or due to the underlying flu. Many of the commoner drug side-effects are similar to symptoms of viral illness (for example – headache, feeling sick, vomiting, diarrhoea, skin rash) so distinguishing them can be difficult.

The researchers received replies on behalf of 43 children aged 4–11 and 60 children aged 11–14 from one primary and two secondary schools that had confirmed cases of swine flu H1N1 in London in April–May 2009. Of these 103 children, 95 had been offered Tamiflu for prophylaxis, of whom 85 (89%) actually took any of the Tamiflu. Just less than half of the primary schoolchildren completed a full course of Tamiflu but three quarters of the secondary schoolchildren completed a full course.

More than half of all schoolchildren taking prophylactic Tamiflu reported one or more side-effects. The most frequently-reported symptom overall was nausea (29%), followed by stomach pain/cramps (20%) and problems sleeping (12%). Gastro-intestinal side-effects (defined as one or more of the following symptoms – feeling sick/nauseous, vomiting, diarrhoea, stomach pain/cramps) were reported by 40%, and almost one in five schoolchildren (18%) reported a 'neuropsychiatric side-effect', such as poor concentration, inability to think clearly, problems sleeping, feeling dazed or confused, bad dreams and nightmares, strange behaviour. A neuropsychiatric side-effect was more commonly reported by secondary (20%) than primary (13%) schoolchildren.

There are a few problems with relying on this research, conducted during a pandemic scare and without a placebo group to compare with. The researchers contacted 256 children but only 103 replied, a response rate of only 40%. When the response rate to a survey is low, this can lead to all sorts of bias in the results. It could be that more of the

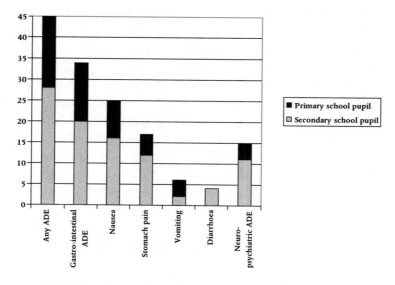

Figure 5. Main symptoms reported by schoolchildren taking Tamiflu in three London schools following contact with confirmed swine flu cases (85 children in total). ADE = Adverse Drug Event.

parents of children who had side-effects responded to the survey, making the drug look worse. Alternatively, if a child was unwell from side-effects, fewer parents might have had the time to respond to an online survey, making the drug look better. The questionnaire was emailed to parents/pupils on the morning of Thursday 14 May 2009 asking for completion by midnight that night so the families had very little time to reply and in some cases were recalling events from weeks previously. Perhaps some of those who reported side-effects experienced them only briefly and were perfectly well after the first dose and happily continued the full course of Tamiflu? Despite the high rate of reported side-effects in secondary school pupils, three quarters of them completed the ten-day course.

The questionnaire prompted parents about specific gastro-intestinal and neuropsychiatric symptoms in their child after taking Tamiflu, perhaps leading to suggestion. The high level of reported side-effects may also have been because the children had high anxiety levels due to the outbreak – nausea, vomiting and not sleeping can all be symptoms of stress. The possibility of group psychological effects (akin to 'mass hysteria') leading to an apparent cluster of symptoms is possible as the children knew one another. If it is rumoured that side-effects are frequent, students may over-report and there is the possibility of 'autosuggestion' through discussion of symptoms on social networking sites such as Facebook.

Another piece of research published in July 2009 described the results of a ten-day course of Tamiflu given to 11–12-year-old pupils in a secondary school in south-west England which was closed for ten days in response to a confirmed case in a pupil. The questionnaire was given to pupils three weeks later, after the school had re-opened. Questions included symptoms of flu-like illness, compliance with taking the drug and side-effects. All 248 children aged 11–12 present on the day (which was over 90% of the whole year group) completed the questionnaire so this is a more reliable survey. Seventy-seven per cent took the full course of Tamiflu and 91% took at least seven days of the ten-day course. Fifty-one per cent experienced symptoms such as feeling sick (31%), headaches (24%) and stomach ache (21%). It is possible that in some instances children may have attributed symptoms that were due to other illnesses to the use of Tamiflu. The reason compliance was high, despite the high frequency of side-effects, may reflect the fact that this was the first school affected by the outbreak in the UK. There was high media attention at the time and reports coming out of Mexico suggested that this novel strain could result in serious disease.

Does giving Tamiflu to childhood contacts prevent flu?

Prior to 2005, there had been one randomized trial of Tamiflu for the prevention of influenza transmission in households (i.e. post-exposure prevention), reporting data from 222 childhood contacts, of whom 129 were in contact with a definite, proven case of flu. In 55 children who had contact with a proven case of flu and were given Tamiflu, only six (11%) developed flu later. In 74 children who had contact with a proven case of flu and were not given Tamiflu, 18 (24%) developed flu later. Therefore the Tamiflu appeared to be effective at reducing the transmission rate from 24% to 11%, preventing spread in 55% of cases. There is a rider to this. The result was not 'statistically significant'. That is, the number of children studied was too small to be absolutely sure that this apparent benefit wasn't just a quirk of chance. But if you were a betting person, the odds look favourable rather than unfavourable.

However, the effectiveness of antiviral prophylaxis is dependent on compliance with taking the medication. In this research trial, compliance was very good with more than 90% of children taking all their drug doses. But this trial was not conducted in the midst of a spreading pandemic and it contrasts with the study of three London schools during April and May 2009 where three quarters of secondary schoolchildren but less than half of primary schoolchildren completed a full course.

Cochrane Review of Tamiflu and Relenza in children

The high rate of reported side-effects in these two 2009 studies contrasts with the findings in a Cochrane review on the use of Tamiflu or Relenza for preventing and treating influenza in children. A Cochrane Review is a piece of research that looks at all the hard evidence worldwide. In this review covering the available evidence up to 2005, the only side-effect that was considered more common with Tamiflu than with placebo was vomiting.

The researchers identified all double-blind, randomized trials comparing neuraminidase blockers with placebo in children less than 12 years of age.

Doctor speak

double-blind = neither the child, the parent, nor the doctor knows whether the child has been given Tamiflu or dummy drug – the researcher knows only when the results are analyzed.

randomized = the decision whether to give the child Tamiflu or a dummy drug is based on the 'toss of a coin'

Three trials involving the treatment of 1500 children with a clinical diagnosis of influenza were included, of whom 977 had laboratory-confirmed influenza.

Side-effect rates in these randomized trials

Researchers tend to talk about 'adverse event' rates rather than side-effects because, as discussed above, it can be hard to know whether a skin rash, say, is due to the drug or the disease the drug is being used to treat. The adverse events rate with Relenza was the same as with placebo. Vomiting was more common in children treated with Tamiflu.

The overall rate of adverse events was similar for Tamiflu and placebo, although children treated with Tamiflu were almost twice as likely to experience vomiting. In one study of Tamiflu in 257 children, none withdrew because they couldn't tolerate the drug. Vomiting occurred in 31 of 158 children who received twice-daily treatment (21%) compared with 10 of 99 children who received Tamiflu once daily (10%).

Less than 1% of patients allocated to Relenza reported nausea, 3% reported vomiting and 1% reported diarrhoea. The rates were very similar in the dummy drug group. More than 97% of children completed eight to ten drug doses.

But this research didn't involve children with the new 2009 swine flu virus?

None of this research involved swine flu. The information we have is based on the use of antiviral drugs to treat children during winter flu. However, there is no reason to believe that these drugs are not just as effective against swine flu which is from the same family of viruses as seasonal influenza A.

The Cochrane Review was updated mid-2009. Again, it only covered information on children under 12 years and confined itself to randomized trials of neuraminidase blockers (drugs such as Tamiflu and Relenza) in children in the community (that is, not admitted to hospital) with seasonal winter influenza. One new study of the treatment of seasonal influenza and two new assessments of the use of antiviral drugs to prevent influenza in household contacts were identified. Again none of these trials tested efficacy with the current 2009 pandemic swine flu H1N1 strain.

By 2009 there had been four randomized trials on the treatment of influenza (two with Tamiflu and two with Relenza) involving 1766 children (1243 with confirmed influenza, of which 55–69% children had proven influenza A). Treatment trials showed reductions in time to resolution of symptoms or return to normal activities, or both, of 0.5–1.5 days. Based on only one trial, Tamiflu did not reduce asthma attacks in children with previous asthma. Treatment was not associated with reduction in overall use of antibiotics. In children with confirmed influenza, treatment with Tamiflu had no effect on the development of ear infections in children aged 6–12 years, but did reduce the rate of ear infections by half from 31% to 15% in children aged 1–5 years. The fact that Relenza had no effect on ear infection rates might be because less inhaled Relenza reaches the bloodstream than Tamiflu, taken by mouth, and therefore the drug does not reach the middle ear.

Finally, Relenza seemed to cause no more side-effects than placebo (dummy treatment) whereas with Tamiflu an additional one in 20 children treated had experienced vomiting. For comparison, in children with flu who did not receive Tamiflu or Relenza, vomiting occurred in 7%, nausea in 3%, and diarrhoea in 7%. The rate of nausea and diarrhoea was not increased by Tamiflu.

By 2009 there had been a total of three randomized trials for post-exposure prophylaxis (one with Tamiflu, two with Relenza) involving 863 children. In 427 children who had contact with a case of flu and were given Tamiflu, only 17 (4%) developed flu later. In 436 children who had contact with a proven case of flu and were not given Tamiflu, 56 (12%) developed flu later. Therefore the Tamiflu appeared to be effective at reducing the transmission rate from 12% to 4%, preventing spread in 66% of cases. The overall rates of transmission to contacts were probably lower in this later review (12% compared to 24% in the untreated contacts in the previous review) because the later review included contact with confirmed and unconfirmed flu cases.

The bottom line is that a ten-day course of post-exposure prophylaxis with Relenza or Tamiflu resulted in an 8% decrease in the rate of influenza illness. With the bigger numbers included in the later review, the result is 'statistically significant' so we can have confidence in it. What this means in practice is that 13 children would need to be treated with a ten-day course of Relenza or Tamiflu to prevent one additional child developing influenza.

The authors concluded that neuraminidase blockers provide a small benefit by shortening the duration of illness in children with seasonal influenza and reducing household transmission. They have little effect on asthma exacerbations or the use of antibiotics. Their effects on the incidence of serious complications and on the current H1N1 swine flu strain remain to be determined.

Summary box — Antiviral drugs

- Influenza may be treated with a group of anti-influenza drugs (oseltamivir = Tamiflu; zanamivir = Relenza).

- Both drugs shorten the duration of illness in healthy children by about one day.

- We know less about how effective they are in 'at risk' children

- Tamiflu also prevents ear infections in children under five years.

- Neither drug caused serious side-effects.

- Antiviral drugs prevent spread of influenza to contacts.

A national prevention or treatment strategy?

First, let me make a distinction between prevention (prophylaxis – pronounced *profilaksis*) and treatment. Although there is some evidence that Tamiflu can prevent the spread of flu from infected children to healthy contacts, the UK has moved from a 'containment' phase to a 'treatment' phase. What this means is that there is now so much swine flu circulating in the population that it is pointless offering antiviral drugs to healthy children who have been in contact with a case of swine flu since they are likely to bump into other cases every day over a period of months. The emphasis now in the 'treatment phase' is:

- Rely on symptoms rather than swabbing to diagnose the virus.

- Stop tracing close contacts of those diagnosed with swine flu.

- Offer antivirals only to those diagnosed with swine flu to shorten the illness (see above).

Shutting schools to reduce the rate of spread remains an option, especially if attack rates escalate very quickly. However, even though children stay away from school, they may still meet in large groups outside school. The virus is likely to be circulating for months over the winter and it is not practical for schools to close for this length of time.

How will I get antivirals for my child?

If your child has flu-like symptoms:

- Read up on swine flu symptoms in Chapter 4 or use the NHS Direct 'swine flu symptom checker' at www.nhsdirect.nhs.uk.

- If you are then still concerned, stay at home and either call your GP or your national helpline for swine flu information (telephone numbers can be found on p.155) (see below for when to choose to call your GP). Either of these will be able to provide a diagnosis over the phone.

- If swine flu is confirmed by telephone, you will be given a voucher reference number entitling you child to antiviral medication.

- Give this number to a healthy friend or relative (a 'flu friend') and ask them to pick up the antivirals for you from a designated local collection centre so that you do not have to leave your child and do not have to take your infected child outdoors.

- In the meantime, follow the advice in Chapter 5 – give paracetamol to reduce fever and pain, encourage your child to drink plenty of fluids and let them rest.

The National Pandemic Flu Service

On the 27 July 2009, the UK government launched The National Pandemic Flu Service – a dedicated website (https://www.pandemicflu.direct.gov.uk) and phoneline (0800 1 513 100) for people to check their symptoms and get a unique number which will give them access to antivirals if necessary. A textphone service is available on 0800 1 513 200 (for people with hearing or speech impairments). (Swine flu information telephone numbers and websites for residents of Scotland, Wales and Northern Ireland can be found in 'Useful Resources' at the end of this book.)

To use this service you will need the following information about your child:

- their date of birth
- their current symptoms
- their history of any serious medical conditions
- their home address including postcode.

You will also need a pen and paper to write down the information which will be given to you.

If your child is thought to have swine flu, you will be given a unique access number and told where the nearest antiviral collection point is. You should then ask a 'flu friend' – a friend or relative who doesn't have swine flu and hasn't been in contact with a case – to go and pick up their antivirals.

Anyone who suspects they have swine flu should not in the first instance go immediately to their GP or Accident and Emergency department.

The government recommends that people should contact their doctor direct rather than using the National Pandemic Flu Service if:

- they have a serious underlying illness
- they are pregnant
- they have a sick child under one year old
- their condition suddenly gets much worse, or
- if their condition is still getting worse after seven days (five for a child).

GP authorization voucher for liquid Tamiflu for children under one year old

Young children are considered to be at particular risk of severe influenza and the complications of influenza. Children under one year old with flu-like symptoms will be seen and assessed by a doctor. Liquid Tamiflu will be supplied at Antiviral Collection Points only upon presentation of this voucher. The voucher is evidence of clinical assessment and indicates the dose of Tamiflu for the identified child.

GP authorization voucher for antiviral medicines for adults and children over one year old

This voucher will be given for Tamiflu capsules for children over one year old and for Relenza by powder inhaler for children over five years old who are able to use the powder inhaler.

Online purchasing

I would warn against buying antiviral drugs from online sources. The WHO estimates that up to half the drugs sold online are counterfeit.

Should I give my child antiviral drugs?

A doctor faced with a symptomatic patient cannot yet predict with certainty the course of their illness and whether or not they will be in the small proportion who may become more seriously ill. Therefore, antiviral medication is still being offered to all those with swine flu symptoms in the UK. Swine flu behaves differently to seasonal flu and past pandemics have hit younger people hardest. However, in the majority of children, swine flu will be a mild and self-limiting illness without complications and the child will recover fully within a week. Whether a parent should take up the offer of antivirals is a trade-off between shortening the illness by one day and reducing the risk of complications and running the risk of mild side-effects. There is no easy answer. However, there are certain high-risk groups where the balance is likely to be in favour of treating your child.

High-risk groups

Some groups of people are likely to be more at risk of serious illness if they catch swine flu and ideally should start taking antiviral medication as soon as they are confirmed with the illness. Antiviral therapy is most effective within 48 hours of symptom onset, and probably has limited value after this time. However, part of the problem for doctors and the public is that the current advice about which groups are at higher risk is still evolving and sometimes contradictory. As of August 2009, the UK government's position is as stated in the box opposite.

The statement that all those with asthma diagnosed in the past three years are at increased risk is contentious. About one in five young children will have had a wheezy episode at some point. I doubt if all of these are at serious risk from swine flu. Children on high doses of steroid inhalers long term may be more vulnerable because of immunosuppression but this is unlikely to be significant at the commonly used doses of 400 micrograms per day or less. The Cochrane Review referred to earlier concluded that there was no evidence of benefit of Tamiflu in those with asthma. From the perspective of pandemic use, however, it should be noted that there was no evidence of harm in this group either.

Who is at risk?

Some groups of people are more at risk of serious illness if they catch swine flu. It is vital that people in these higher-risk groups get antiviral drugs and start taking them as soon as possible – within 48 hours of the onset of symptoms.

Health authorities are still learning about the swine flu virus, but the following people are known to be at higher risk:

- pregnant women
- people aged 65 years and older
- young children under five years old.

People suffering from the following illnesses are also at increased risk:

- chronic lung disease
- chronic heart disease
- chronic kidney disease
- chronic liver disease
- chronic neurological disease
- immunosuppression (whether caused by disease or treatment)
- diabetes
- patients who have had drug treatment for asthma within the past three years.

(www.direct.gov.uk/en/Swineflu/DG_177917)

Tamiflu®

Tamiflu is the common brand name for the antiviral drug **oseltamivir** made by the company Roche. This is a prescription-only medicine available on the NHS for adults and children.

Tamiflu comes in both a gelatine-coated capsule form (capsules come in 30 mg, 45 mg and 75 mg strength) and a liquid suspension which is sugar-free and tutti-frutti-flavoured in a strength of 60 mg/5 ml (contains sorbitol as a sugar-free sweetener). How much Tamiflu to give, how to use the capsules and how to give the NHS alternative to this commercial suspension are all provided in detail below.

Licensed use of Tamiflu

Tamiflu is licensed for adults and children over one year. It is not licensed for use in children under one year because there have been insufficient patient studies evaluating its use in this age group. The leaflet which comes with the Tamiflu might alarm you by saying it should not be given to children under the age of one. However, there is a risk that without giving some guidance, families given Tamiflu to treat older children will also give it to affected siblings under one year in an uncontrolled way. Therefore the doses which are listed in the section below on children under one year have been agreed nationally.

As I noted in Chapter 5, just because a medicine is not licensed for children it does not mean it is unsafe and often we have to make the best recommendation we can with the information available, although ideally we would like to have more information. Doctors prescribing for a child should choose the medicine which offers the best prospect of benefit for that child, even if it is unlicensed. There is published evidence from Japan that Tamiflu has been used safely at a dose of two milligrams per kilogram body weight twice daily in children under one year of age.

Indications and dose for children over one year

Tamiflu is given by mouth. **The dose for *treatment* of flu is twice a day and the dose for *prevention* of flu is once a day.**

Weight	Age if weight not known	Post-exposure Prophylaxis	Treatment of swine flu
Under 15 kg	Over 1 year and under 3 years	30 mg once a day for 10 days	30 mg twice a day for 5 days
15–23 kg	3 years and under 7 years	45 mg once a day for 10 days	45 mg twice a day for 5 days
23–40 kg	7 years and under 13 years	60 mg once a day for 10 days	60 mg twice a day for 5 days
Over 40 kg	13 years and over (including adults)	75 mg once a day for 10 days	75 mg twice a day for 5 days

Administration of capsules

- Give Tamiflu with food (even a snack) as it may reduce the chances of your child feeling or being sick after a dose.

- Toddlers, children and adults will be given capsules. Children younger than five years are unlikely to accept capsules and many older children (and even some adults!) gag when trying to swallow capsules. However, the capsules can be opened and the contents mixed with food. The same applies if people are reluctant to take the capsules because the capsule shell contains gelatin (an animal product, usually from beef). The powder tastes very bitter and experience has shown that, unless the flavour is disguised with blackcurrant juice or chocolate syrup, young children often refuse further doses.

- Infants under one year will not be given capsules but will be given liquid doses (see below).

How parents can best disguise the flavour of Tamiflu capsules

- The capsule can be opened and the powder contents stirred into one teaspoonful of 'squeezy' chocolate syrup (the runny syrup that is poured or squirted over desserts; not chocolate spread) or one or two teaspoons (5–10 ml) of undiluted concentrated blackcurrant drink such as Ribena®. Despite the wording on Ribena labels saying the products are unsuitable for children under three years, if the small amount means children accept their doses of Tamiflu then it can be used. The manufacturer of Tamiflu recommends other foods to disguise the taste, but experience has shown that for young children, undiluted blackcurrant drink concentrate or chocolate syrup work best.

- Thoroughly mix the powder with the syrup or juice – any exposed powder on top of the juice or syrup risks the bitter taste. If the child is due for a dose of paracetamol or ibuprofen syrup then this could be given straight afterwards.

- Try to get your child to swallow all of the mixture. The Tamiflu in the capsule is very soluble and it will dissolve easily so don't worry if there is some powder left over as it not the active part of the Tamiflu drug.

- Do not mix the powder with food or drink in advance; make it up when the next dose is due. Don't leave any 'sitting around'.

Doses for children younger than one year

Children younger than one year can be given Tamiflu but getting the dose right is critical. It should only be given to children under one year in liquid form and the dose depends on your infant's body weight. The recommended dose is two milligrams per kilogram body weight (2 mg/kg – see below for what this means in liquid doses). This is given twice a day for five days for treatment and once daily for ten days for post-exposure prophylaxis. **Note the dose for** *treatment* **of flu is twice a day and the dose for** *prevention* **of flu is once a day.**

Giving these doses to children less than one year

NHS guidance is that the syringe which comes with the commercial Tamiflu solution (12 mg/ml which is 60 mg/5ml in a 75 ml bottle) made by Roche is not suitable for measuring the smaller doses needed for children under one year.

For this reason, in a pandemic the Department of Health has authorized the NHS to produce a solution of oseltamivir supplied with a different oral syringe graduated in millilitres (ml). This NHS suspension will have a different strength of 15 mg/ml. (Note: different strength to the commercial preparation). This will be available in a 20 ml bottle and is referred to as NHS oseltamivir solution below.

So, there are two liquid preparations of oseltamivir that differ in strength. According to NHS Direct, to avoid confusion, under the National Pandemic Plan only the NHS oseltamivir solution (15 mg/ml) will be available from the NHS in the UK. The commercial Tamiflu solution (12 mg/ml) made by Roche should not be available. However, I have provided tables of both doses below in case these arrangements change.

NHS oseltamivir solution: 15 milligrams (mg) per millilitre (ml) in 20 ml bottles specially made by the NHS. The solution is ready to be used and will be labelled with an expiry date of seven days after opening. The solution is not flavoured and has a bitter taste so it is advised to mix the required

LIVERPOOL JOHN MOORES UNIVERSITY
LEARNING SERVICES

dose with one or two teaspoons (5–10 ml) of a concentrated blackcurrant juice such as Ribena. Parents should try to ensure that the child swallows the entire dose. Doses are based on the child's current weight.

Oseltamivir solution 15 mg/ml manufactured by the NHS

Calculation based on 2 mg/kg body weight per dose rounded down to nearest 0.1 ml. Note the dose for treatment of flu is twice a day and for prevention of flu is once a day.

Weight range (kg)	Dose in ml (not mg)
3.0–3.6	0.4
3.7–4.3	0.5
4.4–5.0	0.6
5.1–5.7	0.7
5.8–6.4	0.8
6.5–7.1	0.9
7.2–7.8	1.0
7.9–8.5	1.1
8.6–9.2	1.2
9.3–9.9	1.3
10.0–10.6	1.4
10.7–11.3	1.5
11.4–12.0	1.6

Tamiflu suspension: tutti-frutti flavour, 12 milligrams (mg) per millilitre (ml) in 75 ml bottles made by Roche with an oral measuring syringe. It can be kept at room temperature (25°C, 77°F) for 10 days, or in a refrigerator at 2–8°C for 17 days. The suspension must be shaken before use and should not be frozen.

This suspension is provided with an oral syringe that is graduated in milligrams (mg) rather than millilitres (ml). The lowest measurable dose that should be given with this is 30 milligrams (mg). **It is not suitable for measurement of doses for infants less than one year old.** In circumstances where you have no alternative but to use this Tamiflu suspension for infants under one year, syringes to give liquids in the volumes below into the mouth are available from pharmacists.

Tamiflu suspension 12 mg/ml (60 mg/5 ml) manufactured by Roche
Calculation based on a dose of 2 mg/kg body weight and rounded down to nearest 0.1 ml. Note the dose for treatment of flu is twice a day and for prevention of flu is once a day.

Weight range (kg)	Dose in ml (not mg)
3.0–3.5	0.5
3.6–4.1	0.6
4.2–4.7	0.7
4.8–5.3	0.8
5.4–5.9	0.9
6.0–6.5	1.0
6.6–7.1	1.1
7.2–7.7	1.2
7.8–8.3	1.3
8.4–8.9	1.4
9.0–9.5	1.5
9.6–10.1	1.6
10.2–10.7	1.7
10.8–11.3	1.8
11.4–11.9	1.9
12.0–12.5	2.0

Breastfeeding

The Department of Health for England has decided that Tamiflu is the antiviral of choice for the treatment and prevention of influenza in women who are breastfeeding. Very small amounts pass into the breast milk but not enough to cause concern. Breastfeeding can continue as normal while taking Tamiflu.

Side-effects

Side-effects can include nausea, vomiting, abdominal pain, diarrhoea, headache, conjunctivitis, rash (less commonly). Neuropsychiatric disorders have also been reported.

What if my child is sick (vomits)?

With either capsules or liquid medicine:

- If your child is sick less than 30 minutes after having a dose, wait 15 minutes and give them the same dose again.

- Only repeat the dose once. If your child vomits again, wait until the next dose is due before giving any more. Your capsules or liquid will run out slightly early but don't worry – remember the first 48 hours of treatment are the most important.

- If your child is sick more than 30 minutes after taking a dose, you do not need to give them another dose. Wait until the next normal dose.

What if I give an extra dose by mistake?

Taking one extra dose it is unlikely to do any harm. Your child may feel a bit sick – that is the most common side-effect of Tamiflu.

What do I do if I forget to give my child a dose?

If you forget a dose, do not double the next dose. Take the forgotten dose as soon as you remember and then continue giving doses every 12 hours.

Relenza®

Relenza is the common brand name for the antiviral drug **zanamivir** made by the company GSK.

This is a prescription-only medicine available on the NHS for adults and children five years of age and over who are allergic to Tamiflu or have other reasons which make Tamiflu less suitable (e.g. severe kidney disease). It is taken by inhalation of powder.

Cautions

Avoid in children with asthma.

Dose for children aged 5–18 years (and adults)

For the **treatment of symptoms** in adults and children from the age of five years: two inhalations (2 x 5 mg) twice daily for five days. To be effective it needs to be started within 48 hours of symptoms appearing in adults and 36 hours in children.

For **preventing influenza** in adults and children from the age of five years: two inhalations (2 x 5 mg) once daily for ten days. Therapy should begin as soon as possible and within 36 hours of contact with an influenza case.

Administration

Relenza is a dry powder, diskhaler. Each 'rotadisk' has four blisters and each blister contains the equivalent of 5 mg of Relenza.

Pregnancy

The Department of Health for England has decided that during the swine flu pandemic, pregnant women who are close contacts or have symptoms of influenza should have a course of Relenza rather than Tamiflu because it is inhaled and only low levels appear in the blood.

Breastfeeding

Tamiflu is recommended by the Department of Health for treatment and post-exposure prevention of influenza in women who are breastfeeding. If a woman is prescribed a course of Relenza just before her baby is born she should finish her course of Relenza – there is no need to switch to Tamiflu or stop or delay breastfeeding.

Side-effects

Very rarely Relenza can induce an asthma-like attack of wheezing, or facial swelling, or a rash which may look like nettle stings, or neuropsychiatric disorders.

Ibruprofen, paracetamol and antibiotics are safe to take with Tamiflu and Relenza.

Antibiotics

Antibiotics do not treat viruses. Antibiotics are used to treat swine flu patients who develop certain bacterial complications, such as pneumonia. Antibiotics are available in the UK only by prescription and are not available over the counter or from the National Pandemic Flu Service telephone line (0800 1 513 100).

The NHS already holds substantial stocks of antibiotics and new orders have been placed for over 15 million courses of antibiotics to help in the fight against swine flu.

The government's published advice on the use of antibiotics in children is somewhat contentious. It could be interpreted as recommending that all children who attend hospital with a 'flu-like illness' but are not ill enough to warrant admission should be sent home with a supply of antibiotics – either co-amoxiclav or clarithromycin (if allergic to penicillin).

- *Co-amoxiclav* is a broad spectrum antibiotic from the penicillin family. It contains the more familiar drug amoxicillin with a second drug to reduce the chances of the bacteria being resistant. **If your child is allergic to penicillin, they should not receive co-amoxiclav.**

- *Clarithromycin* is an antibiotic from a non-penicillin family. It has less risk of the side-effects of nausea and vomiting that occur with its older and better known relative – erythromycin (erythroped).

There is no evidence for the recommendation that all children who attend hospital with a 'flu-like illness' but are not ill enough to warrant admission should be sent home with a supply of antibiotics. I do not believe that all children who attend hospital with a 'flu-like illness' but are not ill enough to warrant admission should be prescribed antibiotics. All antibiotics have side-effects and, in some rare cases, these are potentially serious. The widespread use of antibiotics increases the chances of resistant 'super bugs' developing. I think that only children in whom a doctor suspects a bacterial complication of swine flu should be prescribed antibiotics.

When a pandemic of avian flu H5N1 was expected in 2007, the British Infection Society, British Thoracic Society, and the Health Protection Agency in collaboration with the Department of Health published guidelines on the treatment of patients during an influenza pandemic. Although this guidance was intended for bird flu, it is being widely referred to in the current swine flu pandemic. The guidance states that only children who are at risk of complications of influenza, or have a disease severe enough to merit hospital admission during an influenza pandemic, should be treated with antibiotics.

The guidance states that children may be considered at increased risk of complications if they have a cough and a fever greater than 38.5°C, plus either chronic ill health or one of following features:

- breathing difficulties

- severe earache

- vomiting for more than 24 hours

- drowsiness.

These patients should be offered an antibiotic as well as Tamiflu (if over one year of age). The guidance notes that many children admitted to hospital are likely to need oxygen therapy and intravenous fluids as well as antibiotics and Tamiflu.

Two research trials have shown a reduction in the rate of pneumonia and a faster recovery from fever following antibiotic treatment during a seasonal influenza epidemic. One randomized trial of antibiotics in 85 children aged four months to 11 years with influenza-like symptoms during an influenza epidemic showed a decreased rate of pneumonia in the antibiotic treated group (2% versus 16%). There was no change in duration of fever or rate of ear infection. Another randomized trial using two different types of antibiotics in 365 Japanese children with influenza-like symptoms showed faster alleviation of fever (3.8 versus 4.3 days) in the group treated with the erythromycin/clarithromycin type of antibiotic and a decrease in the number of children with chest X-ray evidence of pneumonia (2 versus 13 cases).

Complications of influenza in children treatable with antibiotics

Part of body	Complication	How common?	Comments
Ear	Infection	Very common – 6% overall and up to 30% in children less than 5 years	Treatable with antibiotics
Lungs (Note: the younger the child, the more likely to need hospital admission)	Bronchioloitis	Common	Not treatable with antibiotics
	Viral pneumonia	Common	Not treatable with antibiotics
	Bacterial pneumonia	Common	Treatable with antibiotics
	Croup	Common	Not treatable with antibiotics
Brain	Fever fits	Common	Not treatable with antibiotics
	Coma	Rare	Not treatable with antibiotics
	Guillain-Barre paralysis	Rare	Not treatable with antibiotics
Others	Muscle inflammation	Rare	Not treatable with antibiotics
	Heart inflammation	Rare	Not treatable with antibiotics

The good news is that even in pneumonia, most children do not need intravenous antibiotics. A recent randomized trial comparing oral and intravenous antibiotics in 252 children with pneumonia showed no difference in duration of illness or complications. Oral antibiotics are just as effective and should be given provided that oral fluids are tolerated.

The table on the previous page suggests that only a small proportion of children who have features of swine flu will benefit from antibiotics.

Chapter 7

Swine flu vaccine

How does vaccination work?

Vaccination and immunization are the same thing. Inoculation is another term often used inter-changeably with immunization and vaccination although inoculation literally means the introduction of live, rather than weakened, bugs.

Active immunity means that if we have had an infection once, we cannot (except in special circumstances) catch the identical infection again. So, for example, if you have had chicken pox as a child, when you are an adult you will not catch chicken pox from exposure to children with chicken pox. However, as the common cold, strep throat and influenza demonstrate, there are many infections where the repeat exposure is not to an identical virus or bacterium but to another strain or sub-type and thus re-infection can occur.

Active immunity can be acquired by natural disease or by vaccination. Vaccines stimulate production of antibodies (protein molecules that help our white cells wipe out invading bugs) and other parts of the immune defence system. The principle of vaccination was discovered by Edward Jenner in England in the 18th century. He observed that milkmaids who were exposed to cow pox (not that he knew this was due to a virus) were less likely to get small pox than other family members during a small pox epidemic. He thought that the cow pox somehow conferred protection against the more lethal small pox.

Jenner then undertook the radical step of deliberately infecting James Phipps, a young boy, with pus obtained from a milkmaid with cow pox. James went down with cowpox but was not very ill. Six weeks later, when James had recovered, Jenner infected him with fluid from the sores of a patient with mild smallpox. James did not catch smallpox and 'vaccination' was discovered, the idea of preventing a disease by inoculating a healthy person with a mild infection to prevent a more serious one. Jenner published his findings and called his idea 'vaccination' from the word vaccinia which is Latin for cowpox.

The recognition of germs as the cause of infectious diseases

Almost a century after Jenner's discovery, Robert Koch and Louis Pasteur put forward the 'germ theory' of disease in the 1880s. This was the proposal that micro-organisms caused many human diseases and that these micro-organisms did not appear spontaneously. They opposed the previous theory of spontaneous generation, the idea that living things can arise from non-living things. By dismissing the concept of spontaneous generation, in which disease just happened for no apparent reason, they opened the door to prevention. Perhaps you could somehow prevent yourself catching these tiny micro-organisms? Bacteria had been visualized since the 1670s, first by Anthony van Leeuwenhoek, a Dutchman who perfected the craft of making powerful light microscopes. In 1886, a Scottish doctor called Buist stained the fluid from the skin rash of a smallpox patient with a special dye and saw under the miscroscope 'elementary bodies' which he thought were spores. These were in fact smallpox virus particles, which are one of the only animal viruses just large enough to see with the light microscope.

At the end of the 19th century, in 1892, a Russian botanist showed that extracts from diseased tobacco plants could transmit disease to other plants despite passage of the fluid extract through ceramic filters fine enough to block the smallest known bacteria. The tobacco mosaic virus was the first virus to be discovered. Subsequently, it was proved that viruses could infect animals as well as plants and in 1908 the first virus was discovered which infected humans – poliomyelitis virus.

The body's defences against infection

We now know that all higher animals have a very sophisticated immune system, which is one part of the body's defences to help fight infection. Because of our immune system, humans did not die every time they had an infection even before the era of antibiotics. People survived tooth abscesses, plague, cholera and many other diseases, both mild and serious, although of course the advent of antibiotics increased the chances of survival greatly.

One part of the immune system is made up of white blood cells called lymphocytes. These cells can produce special proteins called antibodies and every antibody is specially made to stick on perfectly to a foreign protein. There is a perfect fit, like a lock and key. Only one key fits each lock and a human measles antibody will only fit onto a measles virus protein. Healthy people don't generally make antibodies against their own proteins (although so called auto-antibody diseases can occur rarely, e.g. rheumatoid arthritis and certain types of thyroid disease). If we did, we would start to attack our own body tissues. But we do make antibodies against anything our body recognizes as foreign, be it an invading bug or a kidney transplant from an unrelated donor. Generally, the production of antibodies is beneficial but in a small minority of people the over-production of antibodies to foreign material such as grass pollen, dog hair or cow's milk protein can lead to allergic diseases such as hay fever, asthma and eczema.

The really clever thing about the immune system is that it can develop an 'immunological memory'. What this means is that if we have been infected with, say, measles once, we can never be infected with it again (unless our immune system is suppressed by drugs or cancer). The next time you are exposed to the measles virus, your body's immune system recognizes and 'remembers' it and rapidly instructs only those lymphocytes with a 'memory' of the measles virus to start manufacturing protective antibodies. Like a homing missile, these lock on to the measles virus which has already entered your body and help destroy it before it can replicate and cause symptoms of infection. The measles virus is wiped out without you even knowing you had it in your body.

Modern vaccination

It was not long before scientists realized that if they could develop an inactive form of a virus, this could be used to fool the immune system into building up a memory without the person ever having to contract the disease. This was an extension of Jenner's idea but instead of using a related virus (cow pox to protect against small pox) to stimulate the immune system, it would be much more effective if they could use the actual virus itself. In the late 1950s, a killed polio vaccine was developed which was given by injection. The recipient of the killed polio vaccine generated antibodies just as if they had suffered a real polio infection, but without the risk of paralysis and death from the real wild live polio virus. Subsequently, a different form of polio vaccine was invented which could be given by mouth on a sugar cube, avoiding the need for a painful injection and expensive syringes in poor countries. This is known as live attenuated polio vaccine (see 'Types of vaccine' below).

The mass vaccination program we now have for children (and travellers) followed. Children can now be protected against a whole range of serious diseases due to viruses and bacteria such as diptheria, tetanus, whooping cough, measles, mumps, German measles (rubella) and some forms of meningitis (due to meningococcal A and C, pneumococcal and haemophilus bacteria). Sometimes a second booster dose of vaccine has to be given to maintain immunity.

Haemophilus influenzae type b (Hib) vaccine

Do not confuse haemophilus influenzae type b (Hib) vaccine with influenza vaccine. Rather confusingly in view of its name, Hib is in fact a bacteria which can cause meningitis. Hib vaccine is not a viral vaccine and has been given routinely to all infants in the UK for over 15 years. It is given by injection at two, three, four and 12 months. It does not protect against swine flu.

Types of vaccine
Vaccines consist of either:

- a *live attenuated* form of a virus (e.g. measles, mumps and rubella vaccine) or bacteria (e.g. BCG vaccine against tuberculosis) – 'attenuated' means weakened: because it is still live, the virus used in a live vaccine stirs up a really good immune response but it has been modified so that it is not able to produce an infection

- *inactivated preparations* of a virus (e.g. influenza vaccine) or killed bacteria (whooping cough)

- *extracts of* or *detoxified poison* produced by the germ (e.g. tetanus toxoid vaccine).

Inactivated vaccines and toxoids may require both an initial series of injections of vaccine to produce adequate protection and one or more boosters (reinforcing injections). For example, in the UK the triple vaccine against diphtheria, tetanus and whooping cough requires three injections at two, three and four months in the first year of life. Diphtheria and tetanus boosters are given again before starting school.

Vaccination against non-pandemic, seasonal flu

Vaccinations against influenza have been developed to protect humans against winter flu. Efforts to limit the impact of influenza on the most vulnerable people are based on widespread annual vaccination campaigns before each winter season. In temperate climates, influenza generally affects people from November to March in the Northern Hemisphere and from May to September in the Southern Hemisphere. It can occur all year round in tropical climates where most of the 500,000 annual deaths occur. Every year strains of influenza (usually type A, more rarely type B) circulate, causing illness in many, hospital admissions for some (mainly older people and young children) and deaths in a minority (mainly in the elderly).

During World War II, a killed-virus vaccine for influenza was developed with backing from the US army. The US army was keen to support this research due to its experience of influenza in World War I, when thousands of troops who had survived the war were then killed by the Spanish flu virus in a matter of months. The most common method of producing influenza vaccine is to grow the virus in hen's eggs, which are used because the flu virus grows well in them and they are cheap and readily available.

- The new virus strain is mixed with a standard laboratory virus strain and the two are allowed to grow together.

- A hybrid forms which contains the inner components of the laboratory strain and the outer proteins of the new pandemic strain.

- The hybrid vaccine virus is injected into thousands of eggs, and the eggs are then incubated during which time the virus multiplies.

- The egg white, which now contains many millions of vaccine viruses, is then harvested and the virus is separated from the egg white.

- The harvested virus is killed with chemicals.

- The outer proteins of the virus are then purified and this becomes the active ingredient in the final vaccine.

An alternative method is to modify the virus so that it loses its virulence and the avirulent virus is given as a live attenuated vaccine (see 'Types of vaccine' above).

The most dangerous side-effect is a severe allergic reaction to either the virus material itself or residues from the hen's eggs used to grow the influenza. However, these reactions are extremely rare.

Four types of influenza vaccine have been developed. The first three are all inactivated and are given by injection. The fourth is live but weakened so it cannot cause serious illness and is given via a nasal spray.

1. Whole virus inactivated vaccines consist of complete viruses which have been 'killed' or inactivated, so that they are not infectious but still stimulate the immune system to produce a response.

2. Subunit inactivated vaccines are made of surface proteins (H and N) only.

3. Split virus inactivated vaccines in which the viral structure is broken up by a disrupting agent. These vaccines contain both surface and internal proteins.

4. Live attenuated, cold-adapted vaccines in which the live virus in the vaccine can multiply only in the cooler nasal passages and which are administered intranasally.

Forms of seasonal flu vaccines

Currently, seasonal flu vaccines are available either as:

- TIV – injection of trivalent (three strains; usually A/H1N1, A/H3N2 and B) inactivated (killed) vaccine, or

- LAIV – nasal spray (mist) of live attenuated influenza virus.

TIV

TIV works by putting those parts of three strains of flu virus into the bloodstream and the body reacting to these by creating antibodies. It has been the most widely-used vaccine against seasonal flu but, because vaccination programs have been targeted only at the elderly, the young and the infirm, the demand for production has been low. As a result, the current worldwide production capacity is for about 500 million doses of trivalent seasonal vaccine per year, less than 10% of the world's population. The process is slow, relying on the growth of that season's most likely strains in eggs and taking up to six months from identification to delivery. About three quarters of the world's seasonal vaccine is produced in Europe and North America and in 2004, when there were production problems at a manufacturing plant in Liverpool, there were fears of a shortage in the US. More than 90% of seasonal influenza vaccine production for the Northern Hemisphere winter (2009–10) was completed by the end of July 2009. Evidence available in September 2009 determines the composition of the Southern Hemisphere's 2010 seasonal influenza vaccine and how much vaccine will be needed.

LAIV

LAIV works by infecting the nose with flu virus that has been modified to minimize symptoms of illness. LAIV is available in the US under the trade name FluMist® and is a vaccine for individuals from two to 49 years of age against the influenza virus subtypes A and type B contained in the vaccine. FluMist should not be given to individuals with previous allergy to eggs, egg proteins, gentamicin, gelatin or arginine, or with life-threatening reactions to previous influenza vaccinations.

FluMist should not be administered to children younger than two years of age due to an increased risk of hospitalization and wheezing which has been observed in clinical trials. Whilst LAIV is not recommended for individuals under age two, it might be comparatively more effective among children over age two – see the Cochrane Review below.

Vaccination strategy against seasonal flu

A vaccine formulated for one year may be ineffective in the following year since the influenza virus changes rapidly and new strains quickly replace the older ones. Influenza viruses A and B (especially A) are constantly altering their protein structure through changes in the haemagglutinins (H) and neuraminidases (N) on the surface of the viruses. It is essential that seasonal influenza vaccines in use contain the H and N components of the prevalent strains recommended each year by the World Health Organization (WHO).

This poses problems for companies manufacturing vaccines and governments buying them, as a new vaccine closely matching the new circulating strains must be produced in time for the beginning of each new influenza 'season'. Every year, the WHO predicts which strains of the virus are most likely to be circulating in the next year, allowing pharmaceutical companies to develop vaccines that will provide the best immunity against these strains.

It is possible to get vaccinated and still get influenza. The vaccine is reformulated each season for a few specific flu strains but cannot possibly include all the strains actively infecting people in the world for that season. As noted above, it takes about six months for the manufacturers to formulate and produce the millions of doses required to deal with the seasonal epidemics. Occasionally, a new or overlooked strain becomes prominent during that time and infects people although they have been vaccinated. It is also possible to get infected just before vaccination and get sick with the very strain that the vaccine is supposed to prevent, as the vaccine takes about two weeks to become effective.

Most developed countries have vaccination programmes covering the elderly and the so-called 'at risk' groups (for example, people with pre-existing conditions or diseases likely to be made worse by influenza infection).

UK recommendations for seasonal flu vaccine in children

Influenza immunization is recommended only for children at high risk. Annual immunization is strongly recommended for children (including infants that were preterm or low birth-weight) aged over six months with the following conditions:

- chronic respiratory disease (includes asthma treated with continuous or repeated use of steroids taken by inhaler or by mouth, or asthma with previous exacerbations requiring hospital admission)

- chronic heart disease

- chronic liver disease

- chronic kidney disease

- chronic disease of the brain, nerves or muscle weakness

- diabetes

- a weakened immune system because of disease (including absence of the spleen or a poorly-functioning spleen e.g. sickle cell disease) or treatment (including cancer drugs and prolonged steroid treatment)

- HIV infection (regardless of whether the child has a weakened immune system or not).

Influenza immunization is also recommended for children living in long-stay facilities and should be considered for household contacts of children with a weakened immune system.

Influenza vaccines for annual immunization in the UK

Almost a dozen different seasonal flu vaccines are available by prescription in the UK. Certain inactivated influenza vaccines are not licensed for use in children under four years but many are licensed down to the age of six months. Those available in the UK use a mixture of the technologies available (e.g. split virus, surface proteins). Up to the age of 13 years, the vaccine injection is repeated a second time after four to six weeks in children not vaccinated before in previous winter seasons. Live attenuated nasal flu vaccine is not prescribable for children in the UK.

Mercury and vaccines

Where possible, children should receive a thiomersal-free influenza vaccine. Thiomersal (also known as thimerosal and mercurothiolate) is a mercury-based substance that is added to some vaccines to prevent them from being contaminated by bacteria and fungi. Thiomersal is also used as an inactivating agent in the very early stages of production of some killed vaccines. Only minuscule amounts of thiomersal used for this purpose remain after the manufacture is completed.

Some seasonal flu vaccines contain thiomersal and some do not. In the past, concerns have been raised over the safety of thiomersal in vaccines. Three studies involving over 600,000 children have examined this issue and all three studies produced very reassuring results. None of the studies found any link between thiomersal exposure from the UK childhood immunization programme and disorders such as autism. Thiomersal is converted to ethyl mercury, whereas the mercury that may be poisonous in the diet is methyl mercury. Ethyl mercury is cleared out of the blood and tissues much more effectively than methyl mercury.

Therefore, if a thiomersal-free swine flu vaccine is not available, a thiomersal-containing swine flu vaccine should be given.

Summary box – Mercury in vaccines

The levels of mercury in vaccines are extremely low and extensive studies in the UK and Denmark have not found any evidence of long term harm, including autism.

The only evidence of harm due to thiomersal in vaccines is a small risk of allergic reactions (skin rashes or local swelling at the site of injection).

What is the evidence that flu vaccines prevent influenza in healthy children?

Children and the elderly are the two age groups that appear to have the most complications following an influenza infection but, until recently, young children were not commonly given flu vaccine. However, for the influenza season 2004–05, the American Academy of Pediatrics and the US Centers for Disease Control and Prevention recommended that immunization of healthy children aged between 6 and 23 months be started as a public health measure. This was later extended to cover children aged 6–59 months. Is this advice justified? A Cochrane Review (see Chapter 6 for an explanation of these reviews) published in 2009 looked at this question. Its findings are explored below.

Previous reviews on the effects of the use of vaccines to prevent influenza in older age groups showed a striking difference between the vaccine efficacy (reduction in number of laboratory-confirmed cases of influenza) and vaccine effectiveness against influenza-like illness (reduction in symptomatic cases), which can include illness caused by influenza viruses that is not laboratory-confirmed or illness caused by other viruses, such as respiratory syncitial virus (RSV).

Fifty-one studies with 294,159 observations were included in this comprehensive review. From randomized trials, live vaccines showed an efficacy of 82% and an effectiveness of 33% in children older than two years compared with either placebo (dummy vaccination) or nothing at all. Inactivated vaccines had a lower efficacy of 59% than live vaccines but similar effectiveness of 36%. In children under two years, the efficacy of inactivated vaccine was no better than placebo.

However, the researchers could not find sufficient data to draw firm conclusions on which vaccine was best or whether one or two dose schedules should be used for inactivated vaccines.

There was only one safety study of inactivated vaccine in children under two years carried out nearly 30 years ago in only 35 children. However, we must set against this the experience in the US of giving influenza vaccine to such young children since 2005. There has been no suggestion of major safety issues in young children.

In contrast, ten studies were found in which the safety of the live attenuated intra-nasal vaccine has been tested in younger children. The authors of the review noted, however, that the manufacturers' refusal to release all safety outcome data from trials carried out in young children makes interpretation of the safety of live attenuated vaccines in this group difficult.

Vaccination during a flu pandemic

Pandemic influenza occurs when a new influenza A virus subtype emerges which is markedly different from recently circulating subtypes and strains, and is able to:

- infect humans
- spread efficiently from person to person
- cause significant clinical illness in a high proportion of those infected.

Because the virus is new in humans, a high proportion of the population will have little or no immunity, producing a large pool of susceptible persons so that the disease spreads widely and rapidly. If a vaccine can be developed quickly enough, this is the best method of preventing cases.

Vaccine against swine flu

The WHO does not expect the swine flu vaccine to be widely available until the end of 2009. Vaccine producers can produce up to a billion doses of any single vaccine each year and as a result WHO anticipates a global shortfall for the world's population of over six billion people. However, if the peak surge does not occur until 2010, the WHO estimates that a maximum of 4.9 billion doses could be produced over a 12-month period if production went well. A more realistic estimate is at least one to two billion doses produced per year. The number of people who might be vaccinated will not be known until it is determined whether one or two doses of the vaccine will be needed to achieve protection and how much viral protein needs to be in each shot.

Although vaccination is a very effective way of preventing disease, it only works if most people are vaccinated. Although, in the worst predictions, 30% of the world's population could be infected with swine flu, no one can predict which people will be in the 30%. The real problem is that enough vaccine may not be available before the surge in cases.

The first batches of vaccine may arrive in the autumn of 2009 and 30 million double doses – enough for half the population – are expected to be available to the UK government by the end of 2009. The UK government has ordered enough vaccine for the whole population and, when it becomes available, will focus first on health professionals and those at the greatest risk.

Which type of swine flu vaccines will be available in the UK?

Nasal seasonal flu vaccine is not currently available to children in the UK. However, the US government has placed a contract with the manufacturer of nasal flu vaccine to see if they can produce an intra-nasal live attenuated HIN1 swine flu vaccine. In the US and the UK there are also well advanced strategies for trials of an injectable inactivated H1N1 swine flu vaccine, first in adults and subsequently in children. It is too early to say precisely what forms of effective swine flu vaccine will become available during the worldwide pandemic and therefore I have covered all options. Furthermore, the Cochrane Review of all information available from seasonal flu vaccination in children included information on both intra-nasal live attenuated vaccines and inactivated vaccines given by injection.

Although most flu vaccines will be produced using chicken eggs, a few manufacturers may culture the virus in vats of cells for vaccine production. This technique would avoid the allergic reactions which can sometimes occur with vaccines produced using eggs and would shorten the production time by about a month. A genetically engineered vaccine (which is available to prevent hepatitis B virus infection, for example) has not yet been developed against flu.

One of the seasonal flu vaccines currently available for people with weakened immune systems contains an 'adjuvant'. Adjuvants are chemicals which help boost the power of inactivated vaccines containing dead organisms or just pieces of the bug or their poisonous chemicals (toxoid vaccines). They have been used for many years and are safe. It is possible the use of adjuvants in a new swine flu vaccine could allow the use of a smaller amount of viral protein in each dose and therefore allow production of more doses worldwide.

When will swine flu vaccine be available?

Making new influenza vaccines generally takes five to six months after first identification of the exact strain of virus. The 2009 pandemic swine flu H1N1 virus was identified at the end of April 2009. The very first doses of swine flu H1N1 vaccine suitable to immunize people, from one or more manufacturers, are expected as early as September 2009. Health-care workers worldwide should be immunized as a first priority although a recent UK survey suggested that a third of nurses would be reluctant to be immunized. This perhaps reflects their assessment that swine flu is a fairly mild illness in most previously healthy people.

High-risk groups

It is especially important that high-risk groups get the vaccine as soon as possible. High-risk groups of children are likely to be similar to those recommended to have seasonal flu vaccine:

- Children with:
  - ◦ asthma or other chronic lung disease
  - ◦ chronic heart disease
  - ◦ chronic kidney disease
  - ◦ chronic liver disease
  - ◦ chronic kidney disease
  - ◦ chronic neurological disease
  - ◦ diabetes
  - ◦ immunosuppression (whether caused by disease or treatment).
- Young children under five years old.

The current seasonal flu vaccine will provide little or no protection against H1N1 swine flu. Nevertheless, it is likely that immunization with the seasonal flu jab will be recommended for high-risk children as well to help prevent them from being infected with both swine flu and this winter's seasonal flu at the same time. Vaccination against seasonal influenza should begin as soon as vaccine is available and before the onset of the winter influenza season. Therefore, two injections may be required for the swine flu and a further two will be needed for seasonal flu to provide maximum immunity in children aged below 13 years who have not received it before.

Although the WHO states that a fully-licensed vaccine might not be widely available until the end of 2009, there will be comparatively little safety data about any rare complications of a swine flu vaccine since any rare side-effects will not show up until millions of people have been immunized. Nevertheless, a number of countries, including Britain, Belgium, Greece, France, Finland, Sweden and the US have already placed orders for the vaccine and are preparing to start mass immunization once it is given approval. This is largely on the basis that previous seasonal flu campaigns have had a good safety record.

Vaccine scares – confusing 'association' and 'causality'

Most vaccine scare stories have arisen because two things happen together but then someone interprets this wrongly as one causing the other. For example, say I tell you that heavy coffee drinkers are more likely to die of lung cancer. A newspaper jumps the gun and runs a headline, 'Coffee causes cancer'. But what if the real reason is that people who are heavy cigarette smokers tend also to be heavy coffee drinkers? You see – coffee and lung cancer happen to be associated but coffee does not cause lung cancer. If A stands for coffee, B is lung cancer and C are cigarettes, then A (coffee drinking) and B (lung cancer) go hand in hand but A does not cause B. The true cause is C which is called a 'confounder'.

Some apparent adverse events of any new swine flu vaccine will be coincidental – that is, occur close in time with vaccine administration, yet are not directly caused by the vaccine. There are lots of examples to illustrate this pitfall. DTP vaccine (diptheria/tetanus/whooping cough vaccines) is given in the UK at two, three and four months of age. Cot death is most common at three to four months of age. People understandably cast around for a reason why their previously well baby suddenly died in the night. If we are vaccinating over 600,000 babies every year in the UK at four months, inevitably some will have had a jab in the week before cot death. That doesn't mean the jab caused the cot death. A and B occur in the same week, but A doesn't cause B. There are lots of other examples. Cerebral palsy is sometimes not obvious before nine months of age, fever fits peak between one and three years of age, autism is often not diagnosed before three years of age, and so on. Parents want a reason why their child, who was apparently a healthy newborn baby, develops problems later and there will always be a high chance of a vaccine in the previous days or weeks to blame.

However, history also teaches us that new vaccines are not without risk. The example below is not written to scaremonger but simply to illustrate.

Will a new swine flu vaccine be safe?
The 1976 US outbreak

On 5 February 1976 an army recruit at Fort Dix in the United States said he felt tired and weak. He died the next day and four of his fellow soldiers were later hospitalized. Two weeks after his death, the cause of death was identified as a new strain of swine flu, a variant of H1N1. It was detected only until 9 February 1976 and did not spread beyond Fort Dix. Nevertheless, it was decided that every person in the US should be vaccinated against the disease. A vaccine was developed and on 1 October 1976 the immunization program began. By 11 October, approximately 40 million people, or about 24% of the population, had received swine flu immunizations. That same day, three elderly people died soon after receiving their swine flu vaccinations and the media immediately linked the deaths to the immunizations despite the lack of positive proof. Subsequently, it was shown that the deaths were not related to the vaccine but it was too late. The US government had long feared mass panic about swine flu – now they feared mass panic about the swine flu vaccinations.

There were also reports of Guillain-Barré syndrome, a temporary paralyzing disorder, affecting some people who had received swine flu immunizations. Guillain-Barré syndrome sometimes develops following a variety of infections, including influenza. It is a rare side-effect of modern seasonal influenza vaccines, with a risk of one to two cases per million vaccinations. However, during the 1976 vaccination campaign there were about 500 cases of Guillain-

Barré syndrome (about ten persons per million vaccinated), resulting in the death of 25 people from weakness of the muscles of breathing. It appeared that the vaccine killed more Americans than the disease. In total, less than a third of the US population had been immunized by the end of 1976 when the National Influenza Immunization Program in the US was halted.

The reason why Guillain-Barré syndrome developed in association with that specific vaccine has never been firmly established and the potential for the development of a similar risk with any future swine flu vaccine can never be firmly excluded. However, the difference this time is that there is already a worldwide pandemic, not a few cases confined to Fort Dix. Thousands of people will die worldwide from swine flu. Even ten persons with Guillain-Barré syndrome (most often a temporary illness) per million vaccinated might be an acceptable price if swine flu could be stopped in its tracks.

It will be interesting to see how the public react to a newly available swine flu vaccine. There is also no evidence to believe that multiple separate injections of vaccine (see above – high-risk children may require up to four jabs) carry any greater risk, although obviously it is unpleasant for children to be needled any more than necessary.

Finally, there remains a concern that the virus could change again and that the vaccines currently under production may not protect against any new variant if it mutates.

General advice on cautions with vaccines in children

Most children can safely receive the majority of vaccines. Vaccination should be postponed if the child is suffering from an acute illness with fever. So they won't get a flu vaccination if they are already showing signs of flu.

Remember, vaccines do not treat a disease. They prevent it but only if the vaccine is given two weeks before contact with an infected person. Do not delay considering vaccination until your child is already ill.

However, it is not necessary to postpone immunization in children with minor illnesses without fever or general upset. Children who just have a runny nose or mild cough can safely be immunized.

Which children cannot have flu vaccines?

This depends on the final version which becomes available for mass vaccination, the method of manufacture, the other compounds contained and whether the vaccines are live attenuated or inactivated. I explain further below.

Children allergic to certain antibiotics

A tiny minority of children are allergic to certain antibiotics. Antibiotics are sometimes used as a preservative in vaccines (e.g. neomycin and polymyxin antibiotics are present in some seasonal flu vaccines). Vaccines should not be given to children who have had a confirmed allergic reaction to a preceding dose of a vaccine containing the same vaccine component such as:

- gelatin
- gentamicin
- kanamycin
- neomycin
- penicillins
- polymyxin B
- streptomycin
- thiomersal.

Children allergic to eggs

Children who have had a previous severe allergic reaction to egg (rash, swelling of the face or difficulty breathing) should not be given influenza vaccine if the virus is grown in hen's eggs. Dislike of eggs or isolated vomiting after eating an egg is not a reason to avoid the vaccine.

Children with weak immune systems

Live attenuated flu vaccines should not be given to children who have a weak immune system:

- children being treated with high doses of steroids or other drugs which suppress their immune system

- children with cancer

- HIV infected children – advice from an expert paediatrician should be obtained (HIV-positive children can receive certain live vaccines).

Live vaccines should be postponed until at least three months after stopping high-dose steroids and at least six months after stopping other drugs which suppress the immune system or generalized radiotherapy (at least 12 months after discontinuing drugs which suppress the immune system following bone-marrow transplantation).

General side-effects of vaccines

Injection of a vaccine may be followed by local reactions such as pain, inflammation and redness at the site (usually upper arm or front of thigh in infants). Gastro-intestinal disturbances, fever, headache, irritability, loss of appetite, fatigue, muscle pain and tiredness are among the most commonly reported side-effects. A tiny number of people may have unforeseen allergic reactions causing difficulty breathing or collapse and although all are extremely rare, this can be fatal (less than one in a million vaccinations).

Premature babies

There is no evidence that premature babies are at increased risk of adverse reactions from vaccines and, indeed, they are often at greater risk from illness.

What about children with epilepsy or neurological problems?

Haven't vaccines in childhood been related to later brain problems? No. There was a scare in the 1970s but this was unfounded. Young children can have a febrile convulsion (a fever fit) from any cause of a high temperature and these often run in families. Perhaps three out of every hundred children will experience one or more fever fits, usually due to a childhood infection causing the fever. However, immunization itself can lead to a high temperature and sometimes a fever fit results. If a child has had fever fits before, there is an increased risk of these occurring during fever from any cause including immunization, but this is not a reason not to have immunization. In children who have had a fit (sometimes called a seizure) with a fever but without other complications, immunization is recommended; see below for advice on the treatment of fever.

When a child has had one or more convulsions without fever (as in epilepsy), and their condition is stable and not deteriorating, immunization is again recommended.

When a child has a stable neurodevelopmental problem (e.g. cerebral palsy or Down syndrome), the child should be immunized according to the recommended schedule.

Where the child's neurological problem is still evolving or the diagnosis is unclear, including poorly-controlled epilepsy, immunization should be deferred and the child referred to a specialist.

What should I do if my baby develops a fever after the flu vaccine?

If fever develops after childhood immunization, the infant can be given a dose of paracetamol. Ibuprofen may be used if paracetamol is unsuitable. Seek medical advice if the fever persists beyond 72 hours after the flu vaccine injection.

PARACETAMOL FOR POST-IMMUNIZATION FEVER IN INFANTS

For post-immunization pyrexia (fever) in an infant aged two to three months, the dose of paracetamol is 60 milligrams. An oral syringe can be obtained from any pharmacy to give the small volume required. If necessary, a second dose can be given six hours later.

IBUPROFEN FOR POST-IMMUNIZATION FEVER IN INFANTS

For infants aged two to three months the dose of ibuprofen is 50 milligrams (on a doctor's advice) as a single dose, which can be repeated once after six hours if necessary. An oral syringe can be obtained from any pharmacy to give the small volume required.

Chapter 8

Preventing the spread of swine flu

When are people with swine flu infectious?

People who contract influenza are infective from 24–48 hours before they develop symptoms until about one week later. Children can be infectious for up to ten days after infection. This explains why it so difficult to contain flu – a person can pass it on even before they know they have it and throughout the illness, although they are most infectious soon after they develop symptoms.

Why it can spread quickly?

Evidence from previous pandemics suggests that one person will infect about two others, and that influenza spreads particularly rapidly in closed communities such as schools or residential homes. International travel and trade probably explain why this pandemic has spread so much faster than the three in the last century.

How does flu spread?

Influenza can be spread in two main ways:

- through inhaling the virus-containing aerosols produced by infected people coughing, sneezing and spitting
- through hand-to-mouth transmission from either contaminated surfaces or direct personal contact, such as a hand-shake.

The swine flu virus is spread in exactly the same way as ordinary colds and flu.

The tiny particles of a flu virus can be spread through the droplets that come out of the nose and mouth when someone coughs or sneezes. A single sneeze releases up to 40,000 droplets.

If someone coughs or sneezes and they do not cover their mouth and nose, those droplets can spread about one metre (three feet). If you are very close to the person you might breathe the droplets in.

If someone coughs or sneezes into their hand, those droplets and the virus within them are easily transferred to surfaces that the person touches.

As the influenza virus can persist outside of the body, contaminated surfaces may have traces of the virus, such as door handles, the TV remote control and computer keyboards.

Viruses can survive for several hours on these surfaces. The length of time the virus will survive on a surface varies, with the virus surviving for one to two days on hard surfaces such as plastic or metal, for about fifteen minutes on dry paper tissues but only five minutes on skin. However, if the virus is present in mucus, this can protect it for longer periods.

If you touch these surfaces and then touch your face, the virus can enter your body through your nose or mouth and you can become infected.

Swine flu cannot be spread by cooked pork products, since the swine flu H1N1 virus is killed by cooking temperatures of

70°C (160°F), corresponding to the general guidance for the preparation of pork and other meat.

Can influenza spread to the unborn baby of a pregnant woman?

During the 1993–94 flu season in the UK, 1659 women who were already at least three months pregnant were recruited to a study of flu. Influenza virus infections were identified in 182 out of 1659 (11%) of these pregnant women. In 138 cases it was possible to test the newborn babies' blood and none had evidence of flu infection from their mother. In 12 infants in whom it was possible to take blood at age 6–12 months, none showed evidence of infection.

There is no reason to think that swine flu should be any different. It is very unlikely the virus would pass from a mother infected during the last six months of pregnancy to her unborn baby. We do know that some viruses can cross the placenta affecting the unborn baby, for example chicken pox and herpes viruses, but this does not seem a major risk with flu viruses.

Preventing spread of swine flu
Coughing and sneezing

It may seem very simple and low-tech but good personal health and hygiene habits are the essence of preventing transmission of the virus:

- frequent hand washing with soap and water, or with alcohol-based hand rubs, is very effective at inactivating influenza viruses

- avoiding spitting

- covering the nose and mouth when sneezing or coughing

- cleaning surfaces regularly using alcohol or disinfectant

- not sharing flannels or towels with an infected person.

You can reduce the chances of spreading flu to others by:

- washing your hands regularly – aim for ten times per day

- always carrying tissues

- using tissues to cover your mouth and nose when you cough and sneeze

- using tissues to cover your child's mouth and nose when they cough or sneeze

- binning the tissues as soon as possible.

The slogan **'CATCH IT, BIN IT, KILL IT'** is a simple way to remember this advice.

The faecal–oral route

If your child's swine flu symptoms include vomiting or diarrhoea, this is another potential way the virus can be spread.

When you flush, germs from the lavatory bowl travel as far as six feet, landing on the floor, the sink and even your toothbrush! Always put the lavatory lid down before flushing. Hands are the biggest spreaders of germs in the home. The kitchen sink contains 100,000 times more germs than a bathroom or lavatory and the average kitchen chopping board has about twice as many faecal bacteria as the average lavatory seat. Studies show that hand washing lowers the transmission of diarrhoea, colds and flu. Wash your hands frequently during the day, using hot water and soap, to prevent spreading germs. Wash them every time you've been to the toilet, changed a nappy or soiled bedding and before

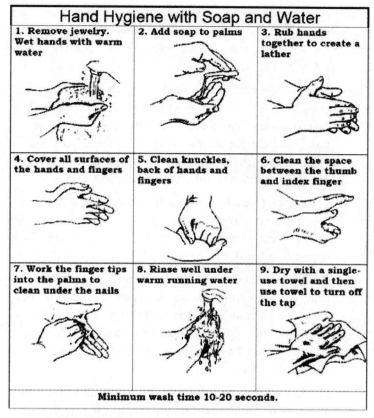

Figure 6. Proper hand washing technique.

and after preparing food. Your child should follow the same rules. Hand washing technique is important – see Figure 6.

Social distancing

This involves staying away from other people who might be infected and avoiding large crowds or perhaps staying home if an infection is spreading in a community. Flu spreads more easily when people congregate close together. This is partly why seasonal flu is confined to the winter months when people spend most time indoors, close together. However, given swine flu will be around for several months, it is impractical for everyone to avoid using public transport over such a prolonged period.

- If you child shows any flu-like symptoms (fever, cough, runny nose), keep them away from nursery or school and avoid contact with other people as much as possible for the next week, especially the vulnerable (other young children, the elderly, people of all ages with chronic health problems).

- Likewise, if you know of a friend, neighbour or relative who is showing any flu-like symptoms (fever, cough, runny nose), keep your child away from them if possible for the next week.

- Build up a network of 'flu friends' (friends and relatives who could help you if you fall ill) and keep their phone numbers nearby. They could collect medicines and other supplies for you or your child so you do not have to leave home and possibly spread the virus.

- Having a stock of food and other supplies available at home that will last for two weeks, in case you and your family are ill. This will avoid you going to the shops and infecting others.

Closure of schools

When swine flu first appeared, there was a policy of closing schools to reduce the spread of infection. When small numbers of people are infected, isolating the sick may reduce the risk of transmission. However, the virus is now so widespread that containment is no longer possible. It is likely the virus will circulate for some months with cases occurring among children in school over an extended period of time. It is not feasible for schools to close for months on end.

During past pandemics, closing schools, churches and other meeting places may have slowed the spread of the virus but did not appear to have a large effect on the overall death rate. Reducing public gatherings, e.g. closing schools and workplaces, may not reduce transmission since people with influenza may just congregate elsewhere.

Masks

The UK Health Protection Agency (HPA) recommends that health-care workers should wear a facemask if they come into close contact (within one metre) of a person with flu-like symptoms to reduce their risk of catching the virus from patients.

This is because any person who is in close contact with someone who has influenza-like symptoms is at risk of being exposed to potentially infective respiratory droplets. In health-care settings, studies suggest that the use of masks could reduce the transmission of influenza.

In the community, however, the benefits of wearing masks has not been established, especially in open areas, as opposed to enclosed spaces while in close contact with a person with influenza-like symptoms. Therefore, the HPA does not recommend that healthy people wear facemasks to go about their everyday business.

Why shouldn't the general public wear facemasks?
Because:
- there is no conclusive evidence that facemasks will protect healthy people in their day-to-day lives
- the virus is also spread by touching infected surfaces
- wearing a facemask only prevents direct transmission when an infected person sneezes mucus into the nose or mouth of another person from close range

- facemasks must be changed regularly as they are less effective when dampened by a person's breath
- people may infect themselves if they touch the outer surface of their mask
- people may infect others by not disposing of old masks safely
- wearing a facemask may encourage complacency
- people need to focus on good hand hygiene, staying at home if they are feeling unwell and covering their mouth when they cough or sneeze.

The World Health Organization (WHO) recognize that some people will still insist on wearing masks or covering their face with a scarf and give the following advice:

- If masks are worn, proper use and disposal is essential to ensure they are effective and to avoid any increase in risk of transmission associated with the incorrect use of masks.

- Place mask carefully to cover mouth and nose and tie securely to minimize any gaps between the face and the mask.

- While in use, avoid touching the mask — whenever you touch a used mask, for example when removing a mask, clean hands by washing with soap and water or using an alcohol-based hand rub.

- Replace masks with a new clean, dry mask as soon as they become damp/humid.

- Do not re-use single-use masks — discard single-use masks after each use and dispose of them immediately upon removing.

Although some alternative barriers to standard medical masks are frequently used (e.g. cloth mask, scarf, paper masks), there is insufficient information available on their effectiveness. If such alternative barriers are used, they should only be used once or, in the case of cloth masks, should be cleaned thoroughly between each use (i.e. wash with normal household detergent at normal temperature). They should be removed immediately after caring for the ill. Hands should be washed immediately after removal of the mask.

Finally, using a mask can enable an individual with influenza-like symptoms to cover their mouth and nose to help contain respiratory droplets, a measure that might reduce spread if the above stipulations are followed.

Airline hygiene precautions

Some airlines have modified their hygiene procedures to try to minimize spread of infection between passengers and to crew on international flights. Some carriers have increased cabin cleaning and allowed in-flight staff to wear face masks.

Countries with very high population densities, such as Singapore and Hong Kong, have been using infra-red thermal-screening cameras on everyone coming into the country, and quarantining those with a fever until proven to be negative for swine flu.

Chapter 9

How dangerous is swine flu?

Most people who have contracted swine flu recover in a week and do not suffer complications, even without being given antiviral medication.

However, it is also true that symptoms of influenza are more severe and last longer than those of the common cold. Most people will recover completely but a minority will develop serious complications (most commonly pneumonia). Influenza can be deadly, especially for the weak, the young and old, pregnant women and the chronically ill. People with a weak immune system (e.g. advanced HIV infection or transplant patients) are also particularly vulnerable to life-threatening complications. According to the World Health Organization (WHO), as of 10 August 2009, 46 of the 53 countries in the WHO European Region had reported over 33,000 laboratory-confirmed cases of H1N1 swine flu virus infection, including 55 fatalities in seven countries: Belgium, France, Hungary, Ireland, Israel, Spain and the United Kingdom.

Swine flu is different from seasonal flu in that most serious illnesses have been in younger age groups, as happened in all three 20th-century influenza pandemics. A fifth of the cases admitted to hospital from mid-July 2009 were children under the age of five years.

An analysis of the first 1000 cases of swine flu in the UK showed a hospitalization rate of around two per hundred people across all ages. About 40% of these hospitalized patients had one of the pre-existing underlying problems recognized to increase risk from seasonal influenza. Asthma was the most common but other examples included liver disease, lung disease, heart disease and diabetes. According to a WHO report, almost half of 45 fatal cases in Mexico had underlying risk factors including pregnancy, asthma, other lung diseases, diabetes, obesity, poor immune systems, nerve or brain disorders and heart disease.

Serious swine flu cases in UK week ending 15 July 2009

Age group	Under 5 years	5–15 years	16–64 years	65+ years	Total
In hospital	134	84	354	80	652
In intensive care	9	5	29	10	53
Percentage in intensive care	7%	6%	8%	12.5%	8%

It is important to keep these figures in context. There are about 12 million children in the UK of whom over three million are under the age of five years. Therefore, at this time, the numbers of children developing swine flu serious enough to warrant hospital admission are tiny and the proportion requiring intensive care is no greater than for older age groups. A total number of hospital admissions of almost 700 is also very small given that at this time the consultation rate with flu-like symptoms was running at 700 per million of the population per week or about 40,000 consultations per week for the whole of the UK. According to the Health Protection

Agency, at this time five- to fourteen-year-olds were the group predominately affected by the illness in the community with four times as many seeking the advice of their GP compared to other age groups.

Deaths from swine flu in children

By mid-July 2009, there had been 29 deaths in the UK attributed to swine flu, of whom four were children. For each of these families, this is a tragedy. But it is important to keep these figures in perspective. Three of these children had other underlying health problems, which may have made them more vulnerable, and only one was previously healthy. This was a six-year-old girl in whom post-mortem examination revealed both swine flu and blood poisoning (septicaemia) with bacteria called group A strep. Such a septicaemia can kill previously healthy children even in the absence of swine flu. It is impossible to say whether swine flu contributed to her developing the bacterial septicaemia but it is possible – bacterial infection as a complication of swine flu is a significant cause of death from this viral infection.

As a parent, how should you try to differentiate septicaemia from swine flu? In Chapter 4 (p.43) I list the features which if present in your child should lead to urgent hospital referral. Those features don't prove that your child definitely has septicaemia. Ultimately this requires a blood test and a 48-hour wait for the results for proof one way or the other (if bacteria are present in the blood, it may take up to 48 hours for the bacteria to grow to detectable levels in the lab). But your child can be carefully assessed and if there is any uncertainty, antibiotics can be given for 48 hours as a precaution until the blood results are known.

Part of our difficulty in dealing with even a small number of deaths is that fatalities in children from infection have become very rare. In my grandparents' era, almost everyone seemed to have a relative who had died young, perhaps from pneumonia, diphtheria, scarlet fever, peritonitis from a burst appendix or puerperal fever after childbirth. Infections we hardly hear of now. Death rates have been falling in children for over 50 years. The advent of widespread immunization and the availability of antibiotics have made death from infection rare although of course bacterial meningitis remains a killer disease in children. But deaths from viral infections are now incredibly uncommon in developed countries. In 2007, there were two deaths from chicken pox and two deaths attributed to influenza among over 700 deaths in children aged between five and fourteen years. These children may also have had other health problems. These are far out-numbered by the one quarter of deaths due to accidents and one quarter to cancer.

However, whilst the 20th century witnessed remarkable advances in the conquest of killer diseases such as smallpox and poliomyelitis, during the second half of the century new infectious diseases emerged. With the increase in international trade and travel and changes in human lifestyles (for example, greater human–animal contact), new infections have arisen and spread much more rapidly around the world. The onset of HIV in the 1980s and the outbreaks of SARS and avian influenza in the 1990s are examples.

A second reason for our difficulty in coming to terms with something like swine flu is that, whilst we know that preterm and newborn babies are fragile and at risk from disease, we have become accustomed to most children surviving their school-age years. Of all deaths in children aged 0–14 years, 70% occur within the first year of life, 46% within the first month and 35% within the first week. Put another way, the risk of death in the UK drops to around 27 per 100,000 children aged 1–4 and to 12 per 100,000 aged 5–14 compared to a risk of death in the first year of life of 580 per 100,000 live births. Death rates then begin to rise again after the age of 15, particularly in boys and largely as a result of the increasing risk of deaths from accidents.

There have been about 500 deaths out of the first 100,000 confirmed swine flu cases worldwide, a death rate of 1 in 200. This is likely to be an over-estimate since only the more serious cases will have come to medical attention or justified swabbing for laboratory confirmation. A case fatality for swine flu of between 0.1 and 0.4% (1 per 1000 to 4 per 1000) is often quoted. So, even at a conservative estimate of one death per 1000 cases (100 deaths per 100,000 cases), this represents a fatality rate eight times higher than we currently expect for children aged 5–14, which is approaching the rates during my grandparents' childhood at the end on the 19th century.

These estimates of case-fatality rates of 1 per 1000 to 4 per 1000 cases must be treated with great caution. They must also be viewed in a population context. This is the percentage of cases who might die, not the percentage of the population. That depends on the scale of the problem (the 'attack rate' – see below). In a review of influenza-related mortality from the

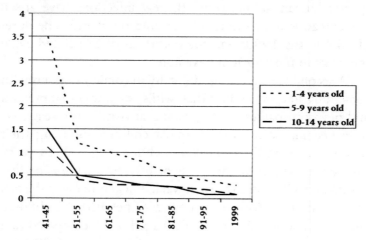

Figure 7. Death rates per 1000 children in the UK from World War II until 1999. There has been little change since 1999.

surveillance of seven seasons (1974–81) of seasonal influenza in Texas, there were large enough numbers during the 1977–78 epidemic to estimate mortality rates. From the table below it can be seen that, even in an epidemic year, the number of deaths was very small and far less common in children than the elderly.

Death rates during a pandemic are determined by four factors:

1. The number of people who become infected – so far fairly low.

2. The virulence of the virus – so far apparently mild.

3. The underlying health of affected populations – people are living longer than ever and nutrition and protection by immunization is better than ever. For example, rheumatic heart disease was a major risk

Harris County Texas, 1977–78 influenza epidemic.

Age	Population	Number hospitalized	Hospitalization rate per 100,000 children of that age attributed to influenza	Deaths	Death rate per 100,000 children of that age attributed to influenza
Less than 1 year	44,000	575	1300	6	14
1–4 years	166,000	552	330	0	0
5–19 years	670,000	401	60	6	1
Over 65 years	128,000	1507	1170	240	187

factor for death in the 1957 pandemic but is almost unknown now in developed countries.

4. The effectiveness of preventive measures — we don't know yet how soon an effective vaccine will be available.

Accurate predictions of mortality cannot be made before the extent of the pandemic is clearer. All estimates of the number of deaths in the initial stages are purely speculative. However, the UK government's advice to a House of Lords Committee in 2008 was sobering:

> 'While there has not been a pandemic since 1968, another one is inevitable, whether or not it arises from H5N1 (bird flu). Estimates are that the next pandemic will kill between 2 million and 50 million people worldwide and between 50,000 and 75,000 in the UK.'

The scale of the problem

An even bigger problem, and what we just don't know at this time, is how many children will be affected overall — the 'attack rate'. If the worst case scenario estimate of a 30% attack rate comes true, then four million children will be infected in the UK. This would lead to 4000 deaths if the fatality rate was 1 per 1000. Even at a conservative estimate of only 5% of all children being infected, this would mean 600,000 UK children infected and 600 deaths if the fatality rate was 1 per 1000.

We have to be very cautious about considering even a fatality rate of 1 per 1000. Apart from the problem of over-estimating the risk because mild cases don't come to attention, the death rate could be much less for the following reasons:

• Tamiflu makes the illness less severe.

• Antibiotics reduce the severity of bacterial infections.

- An effective vaccine may be widely available by the end of 2009.

- Modern intensive care facilities are superior to any which existed during previous pandemics.

What are the main complications of influenza?

Complications arising from infection with influenza are:

- pneumonia
- bronchitis
- sinus infection
- ear infections
- dehydration from excessive vomiting and diarrhoea.

During winter flu epidemics, children under the age of six months are the most likely to be hospitalized. Children with chronic medical conditions (asthma, heart disease, lung disease, weak immune systems, cancer, kidney disease, sickle cell disease and diseases of the brain and nerves) and those born prematurely were 4–21 times more likely to be hospitalized with respiratory complications than healthy children during influenza seasons.

Rarer complications such as myocarditis (inflammation of the heart muscle), myositis (inflammation of the muscles), polyneuritis (inflammation of the nerves causing weakness) and encephalitis (inflammation of the brain) have already been seen in childhood cases of swine flu, albeit rarely.

The most common cause of death due to flu is respiratory failure, either from a direct effect of severe swine flu viral pneumonia or due to a secondary bacterial pneumonia. Overwhelming pneumonia, which limits the ability of the lungs to get oxygen into the bloodstream, can be combated by the use of machines to assist the work of the lungs. The common form is a breathing machine called a ventilator which acts like a bellows, forcing air enriched with high levels of oxygen into the lungs.

In the most severe cases, a type of heart–lung bypass machine (using similar technology to that employed to keep a person alive when their heart is stopped during heart surgery) called ECMO may also help. ECMO stands for Extra-Corporeal Membrane Oxygenator, meaning the blood is diverted from the body to a machine containing very thin membranes where oxygen is mixed with the blood before returning the blood to the body.

One of the most common germs which can cause bacterial pneumonia in flu is called streptococcus pneumonia (pneumococcus). There are vaccines available against many of the pneumococcal strains and these are routinely offered to young children in the UK – make sure your child is up to date with all their immunizations now.

Is it possible to give swine flu vaccine simultaneously with other vaccines?

Inactivated influenza vaccine can be given at the same time as other injectable non-influenza vaccines but the vaccines should be administered at different injection sites. So if your child is coming up for their routine vaccines, they don't need to miss out on those.

Intensive care facilities in the UK

There are currently between 300–350 staffed paediatric intensive care beds in the UK. In addition, there are over 3000 adult intensive care beds. Paediatric ECMO is provided nationally by four centres – London, Leicester, Newcastle and Glasgow.

In a pandemic situation with very high attack rates, paediatric high dependency and intensive care beds are likely to fill quickly and could be insufficient to meet demand. Children may have to be selected for intensive care on the basis of the severity of the child's disease and the likelihood of the child achieving full recovery.

However, there are reasons to be more optimistic:

- Not all children will become ill at the same time – the pandemic is likely to spread over months.

- The number of intensive care beds actually available is greater provided more staff can be recruited to nurse and care for the children in those beds.

- In an emergency, children could be cared for in an adult intensive care unit if there are more severely affected children than adults.

- For previously healthy children, swine flu should be a relatively short illness and most children will respond to therapy, recover and hence free up an intensive care bed.

- Planned, complex surgery (so called elective or 'cold' cases) which would require an intensive care bed for post-operative recovery can be deferred until after the pandemic.

The more pessimistic prediction would be that if 30% of medical and nursing staff are ill, there will be fewer staff to care for sick children.

Living with risk

Living with risk is very tricky but part of life. Doctors use terms like 'rare', 'common', 'unlikely', 'probable' and 'significant' all the time but research has shown that people place their own interpretation on these words – sometimes

Summary — Risk and living with uncertainty

Positives:

- Low attack rate so far.
- Small number of fatalities so far.
- Most will recover at home.
- Anti-viral drugs available.
- Vaccine likely to be available.

Potential unknowns:

- Attack rate may increase during the winter.
- Virus could become more virulent.
- If 30% of population affected, there may not be enough beds for those who need hospital admission.
- Virus could mutate and become resistant.
- Vaccine may not be widely available in time.

people hear what they want to hear. We sometimes have an unrealistic view about relative risks. In the UK each year, horse riding causes about ten deaths and more than 100 road traffic accidents. There are about 30 deaths per year among Ecstasy users. Should the UK ban horse riding? First cousins who marry have three times the risk of having a child with a severe abnormality. Should society ban first cousin-marriages?

In thinking about swine flu and the treatments available, the decision on whether to give your child a treatment needs to balance:

- What is the risk of getting the disease?
- How serious is the disease?
- How much is the risk reduced with treatment?

- What are the risks or side-effects in taking the treatment?

I hope this chapter and others help you explore these risks in a balanced way. Ultimately, it is an individual decision.

Are there any lasting effects of swine flu?

I have mentioned complications of swine flu which occur at the same time as the illness (see above and Chapters 5 and 6). Are there are ever any lasting side-effects? The vast majority of children, even those with severe influenza, make a full and complete permanent recovery. For a small number, there are long term problems – not as a result of the swine flu persisting in the body as some viruses can do, but as complications of the illness. For example, most children who are so severely ill that they need the support of a breathing machine are likely to survive but some may suffer permanent damage to the lungs. Sadly, some of the children who survive encephalitis (brain inflammation) will develop epilepsy or have learning difficulties on returning to school. The rate of these more severe outcomes of influenza, such as encephalitis are likely to be very low.

Final word

For the majority of children, swine flu is a mild illness. Most children who have contracted swine flu recover within a week and do not suffer complications, even without being given antiviral medication. They return to normal activities and suffer no long term consequences. Parents can do a great deal to help their child through swine flu – go back to Chapter 5 to see just how much you can do.

Chapter 10

Frequently asked questions

About the swine flu virus

Q: **What is swine flu?**
A: It is an infectious respiratory disease of pigs caused by type A influenza viruses. Pigs are hit by regular outbreaks. In April 2009 a novel flu strain appeared that combined genes from human, pig, and bird flu viruses. Initially called 'swine flu' this emerged in Mexico before spreading to the United States and then around the world. The World Health Organization (WHO) officially declared the outbreak to be a 'pandemic' on 11 June 2009.

Q: **How do humans catch it?**
A: Humans pass it to each other and it spreads in the same way as seasonal flu – mainly through coughing and sneezing.

Q: **Could my child just get ordinary flu?**
A: Yes but the illness will look very similar and Tamiflu® will still give benefit. So no harm will be done. Your child could be unlucky and get both.

Q: **Are there any lasting effects of swine flu?**
A: The vast majority of children, even those with severe influenza, make a full and complete permanent recovery. Very occasionally, as with any other serious illness, swine flu may lead to later long-term problems.

Q: If my child gets ordinary flu, will they be immune to swine flu afterwards?
A: No. An infection with one strain of flu does not protect against a different one.

Pandemics

Q: What is a pandemic?
A: If the flu spreads over a wide geographic area and affects a large proportion of the population it goes beyond an epidemic and becomes described as a pandemic.

Q: Is the UK especially affected?
A: Initially the outbreak in the UK was far more extensive than in other European countries with the UK having ten times more swine flu cases than anywhere else in Europe during the first months of the outbreak.

Q: Why did this happen?
A: The UK is a hub for international air travel and also millions of Britons now regularly go on holiday abroad. Parts of the UK have a very high population density with people living very close together – ideal conditions for a new flu virus to spread.

Q: How many people will be infected at one time in the UK?
A: It varies from week to week. For example, there was a huge surge in the number of consultations of people complaining of influenza-like illness in the first three weeks of July 2009 in the UK – up from a rate of about 15 people per 100,000 per day to more than 40 per 100,000 per day.

Q: How many people could die in the UK?
A: Sir Liam Donaldson, the Chief Medical Officer for England, presented best and worst case predictions. At best, he estimates that 5% of the population will be infected and 3,100 will die. At worst, if 30% of the population is infected, 65,000 people could die with an overall fatality rate of 0.35% of affected people. In the 1957 flu

pandemic 33,000 people died in the UK and in the 1968 pandemic 30,000 died. In those outbreaks 25–30% of the population was estimated to be infected and the fatality rate was 0.2–0.25% of affected people.

Q: Can the NHS cope?

A: Even though swine flu is no more lethal than ordinary flu and the vast majority of those infected will suffer only mild illness, serious cases could overwhelm the NHS. It has only 3636 intensive care beds, and a third of those are for specialist treatment such as burns and spinal injuries. Though not all severe swine flu cases would arrive at once, even the Cabinet Office admits the intensive care system might struggle to cope. It suggests that 0.5% of clinical cases may require intensive care 'if the capacity exists'. Under such an assumption, if one million people were infected, 5000 would require intensive care.

Q: What are the symptoms?

A: The symptoms of swine influenza in people are similar to the symptoms of the usual seasonal influenza infection. These include sudden onset of a high temperature (over 38°C), fatigue and aching muscles, headache, coughing, runny nose and sore throat. Some people with swine flu will also have vomiting and diarrhoea.

Q: What if my child doesn't have a fever. Can he or she still have swine flu?

A: Yes. Most infected people have a temperature but a minority do not, at least initially, even though this is usually a hallmark of flu. However, they may still be infected.

Q: Are the young being particularly affected?

A: Yes. The groups with the highest rate of flu-like illness are, in order, those aged 5–14, then 1–4 and then 15–24.

Q: How long does swine flu last?

A: How long your child is ill for will depend on the severity of the infection and whether they have any underlying, pre-existing diseases. The average is four days.

Q: Is it safe to travel?
A: The World Health Organization is not recommending travel restrictions. Limiting travel and imposing travel restrictions would have very little effect on stopping the virus from spreading and it has already been confirmed in many parts of the world anyway.

Household 'cough and cold' remedies for swine flu

Q: Can I give my child aspirin?
A: Aspirin should be avoided if possible. Aspirin should never be given to children under 16 years because of the risk of causing the potentially fatal Reye's syndrome.

Q: So what should I do if I think my child has swine flu?
A: If your child feels unwell with a high fever, cough or sore throat:

- keep them at home, away from school and other people
- encourage rest and plenty of fluids
- cover their nose and mouth when coughing and sneezing and, if using tissues, make sure you dispose of them carefully. Clean your hands immediately after with soap and water or cleanse them with an alcohol-based hand rub
- if you do not have a tissue close by when they cough or sneeze, cover their nose and mouth as much as possible
- inform family and friends about your child's illness and try to avoid contact with other people.

Q: Are there any medicines I can give my child without a prescription?
A: You can give paracetamol or ibuprofen as a pain reliever for aches, pains and to reduce temperature (see Chapter 5).

Q: How much fluid should my child be drinking in 24 hours while she is ill?
A: Young babies: around 150 ml (5 fl oz) per kg (2.2 lb) of body weight.

Children less than 10 kg: 100 ml (3–4 fl oz) per kg (2.2 lb) of body weight.

Children more than 10 kg: 100 ml (3–4 fl oz) per kg (2.2 lb) of body weight for the first 10 kg; 50 ml per kg for the next 10kg; and only 20 ml per kg thereafter. (For more information see Chapter 5.)

Q: My child feels sick when he drinks liquids – how do I keep him hydrated?
A: The secret is 'little and often'. Giving a child their recommended fluid intake in teaspoonfuls (a teaspoonful is 5 ml) every quarter of an hour means the liquid is more likely to stay down than offering a large volume in a bottle every hour.

Antiviral medicines

Q: Should I give my child Tamiflu?
A: Yes. Nobody knows at the beginning of an illness how serious flu will be in that individual child. Tamiflu works only if given within the first 48 hours. So start it as soon as possible. Side-effects are uncommon and mild according to the best research studies.

Q: What are the side-effects of Tamiflu?
A: Flu causes vomiting in about 1 in 20 children. If children with flu are treated with Tamiflu, about 2 in 20 children will vomit. This is the only common side-effect.

Q: How do I get Tamiflu for my child?
A: You can telephone a call centre (see 'Useful Resources' for phone numbers in different parts of the UK) or log on to a website (www.pandemicflu.direct.gov.uk) to be diagnosed and prescribed Tamiflu without going through your GP (unless your child is aged under one year when they should be seen by a doctor). A trained call handler will issue you with a reference number if they think your child has swine flu. The website allows computerized diagnosis and will also issue a reference number. Healthy people have been warned that if they successfully fake a diagnosis, it will be hard to get a further dose.

Q: Where do I collect the Tamiflu from?

A: The call handler or website will tell you the nearest collection point. Get a 'flu friend' who is well and has not been in contact with flu to take the child's reference number to a local collection centre (set up in community centres and pharmacies across the country).

Q: How does Tamiflu work?

A: It blocks chemicals on the surface of the virus which hinders it reproducing. That is why it is important to start the course of Tamiflu as soon as possible after the onset of symptoms. It does not cure the illness, but it does reduce its duration and severity. It reduces the length of time children are ill by about a day and reduces the chance of passing on an infection.

Q: Should I give my child antiviral medicines now just in case he or she catches the swine flu virus?

A: No. You should only give your child an antiviral, such as Tamiflu, if you are advised to do so. Antiviral medicines have no long lasting effect so giving your child a course now won't protect them next week and you don't want to keep giving them repeat courses. Individuals should not buy medicines to prevent or fight this new influenza without a prescription and they should exercise caution in buying antivirals over the Internet.

Q: What is the difference between Tamiflu and a vaccine?

A: Tamiflu is an antiviral drug taken by people who already show signs of swine flu. It helps ease your child's symptoms. A vaccine is given before people are infected to reduce their chances of catching the disease.

Q: What does Tamiflu look like and how do I administer it?

A: Tamiflu comes in capsule and liquid preparations and is taken orally. The capsules can be swallowed whole or they can be opened and the contents mixed with food or drink to mask the taste. Liquid Tamiflu is given to babies as smaller doses can be dispensed with a special syringe. (For more information see Chapter 6.)

Q: Is Tamiflu the only antiviral medicine available?
A: No. Relenza®, a prescription-only medicine, is available on the NHS for adults and children five years of age and over who are allergic to Tamiflu or have other reasons which make Tamiflu less suitable (e.g. severe kidney disease). It is taken by inhalation of powder.

Q: Can antibiotics be used to treat swine flu?
A: Antibiotics don't work against any virus, including swine flu virus. Antibiotics are used to treat swine flu patients who develop certain bacterial infections as a complication of the swine flu. Overuse of antibiotics can allow 'super bugs' to develop and all antibiotics have side-effects that can be potentially serious, so only children in whom a doctor suspects a bacterial complication of swine flu should be prescribed antibiotics.

Swine flu vaccine

Q: Should I give my child flu vaccine?
A: Yes. Before the government releases the vaccine for general use all of the data will have been scrutinized by the Joint Committee on Vaccination and Immunization. This is a group of expert scientists with a wealth of experience who are not members of the government. If they recommend it for children, then, as best they can tell, it is safe. Previous flu vaccines have been generally safe in children although they don't seem to work well in children under two years.

Q: When will a vaccine be available?
A: Britain is expected to have received vaccines for half the population by the end of 2009, with the second half expected in 2010. At the moment, children, pregnant women, those with underlying health conditions, the elderly and NHS staff are likely to receive the vaccine first.

Q: How many injections of vaccine will my child need?
A: Experts believe two doses will be necessary to give the most protection against the virus. However, if a particularly potent vaccine is created many people at low risk may be given just one.

Q: Will there be side-effects from the vaccine?
A: All vaccines have some side-effects, although improvements in recent decades mean adverse reactions are expected to be rare and mild.

Q: What can be done to prevent the infection?
A: Cover your or your child's nose and mouth when coughing or sneezing, dispose of dirty tissues promptly and carefully, wash hands frequently (ten times per day) with soap and water and wash cleaning surfaces which are regularly touched. Avoid people with obvious symptoms.

Q: Should I take my child to the doctor?
A: No, unless your child is aged under one or you think they have an illness other than swine flu or they have serious features (see Chapter 4). Doctors don't want potential virus-carriers in their surgeries in case they infect people already weakened by other illnesses. The same goes for hospital Accident and Emergency Rooms.

Q: Should I stop breastfeeding my child if I am ill with swine flu?
A: No. Breastfeeding is protective for babies against viral infections – it passes on helpful ready-made antibodies from the mother which work right away and lowers the risk of respiratory disease. Breastfeeding provides the best overall nutrition for babies and increases their defences against illness.

Q: Is it safe for my child to receive the swine flu vaccine at the same time as other vaccines?
A: Yes. It can be given at the same time as other injectable non-influenza vaccines, but the vaccines should be administered at different injection sites. So if your child is coming up for their routine vaccines, they don't need to miss out on those.

How dangerous is swine flu?

Q: How dangerous is it?
A: In the majority of children it is a mild illness and they make a full recovery. Of confirmed laboratory cases of all ages, about 1 in 200 have died but there are good reasons why this is probably an over-estimate and the true case-fatality rate is probably far lower.

Q: What risk factors make someone more vulnerable?
A: Conditions that make a person more vulnerable to the virus are diseases of the lung (including asthma), heart, kidney, brain or nerves, diabetes, cancer, HIV. In early analyses of deaths from swine flu, obesity came up as a risk factor too.

Q: Do all those admitted to hospital have existing health problems that made them vulnerable?
A: By the end of August 2009, about 40% of people admitted to hospital had pre-existing ill health. In the 1977–78 influenza epidemic, the figure was similar, about 30%.

Q: Have all those who have died had existing health problems that made them vulnerable?
A: The vast majority have but even in ordinary seasonal flu outbreaks a few healthy people may die. In 2003 an outbreak of the H2N3 strain led to the deaths of 17 people aged under 18 even though none of them was considered to be in an 'at risk' group.

Q: Is the virus getting more deadly?
A: No – at least, not yet. At present, swine flu is no worse than ordinary flu but it is likely that many more people will be infected than in an average winter flu season. So more people will be ill and therefore more people will die than in a non-pandemic year.

Q: Can I catch swine flu from eating meat?
A: No, the virus cannot be transmitted by eating foods. Cooked pork products are safe to eat because cooking temperatures kill the virus.

Q: Will wearing a surgical mask prevent me from getting swine flu?

A: There is no conclusive evidence that facemasks will protect healthy people in their day-to-day lives because wearing a facemask only prevents direct transmission from close range. Masks also become less effective quickly when dampened by a person's breath and can harbour the virus, causing infection in the wearer and others if not disposed of correctly. However, the UK Health Protection Agency recommends that healthcare workers should wear a facemask because of their close contact with patients.

Q: How long can the virus survive on surfaces?

A: The virus can stay alive for one to two days on hard surfaces such as plastic and wood, for around 15 minutes on dry paper tissues, and for about five minutes on skin.

Q: Should I keep my child away from public places during the pandemic?

A: If your child shows any flu-like symptoms, keep them away from nursery or school and avoid contact with other people as much as possible for the next week. However, it is impractical to keep a healthy child isolated for the course of a pandemic. In fact, since the outbreak of the pandemic, the UK has moved from a 'containment' phase to a 'treatment' phase, which means schools, churches, etc. are remaining open.

Useful Resources

I have confined the list below to websites that I have personally visited, found to be useful and which are written by credible organizations. Websites have an annoying habit of changing their exact address. If the address given below does not take you there directly, use an internet search engine.

In alphabetical order:

Centre for Disease Control, USA

www.cdc.gov/h1n1flu

Chief Medical Officer for England

www.dh.gov.uk/en/Aboutus/MinistersandDepartmentLeaders/
ChiefMedicalOfficer/DH_19

Health Protection Agency for weekly updates

England: www.hpa.org.uk

Scotland: www.hps.scot.nhs.uk

Wales: Welsh Assembly Government: http://wales.gov.uk/topics/health/
protection/communicabledisease/swine/advice/professional

Northern Ireland: Department of Health, Social Services and Public
Safety: http://www.dhsspsni.gov.uk

Medicines information leaflets

Information for parents:
www.medicinesforchildren.org.uk

NHS Direct factsheets on antiviral drugs:
www.nelm-web.lbi.co.uk

NHS

www.nhs.uk
www.pandemicflu.direct.gov.uk
www.nhs.uk/Conditions
www.immunisation.nhs.uk/files/thiomersalfsht.pdf

NHS Choices

www.nhs.uk/Conditions/Pandemic-flu/Pages/Otherlanguages.aspx
Pandemic Flu information in other languages and formats.

www.nhs.uk/Pages/HomePage.aspx
The health encyclopaedia, common health questions and local services search.

NHS Direct

www.nhsdirect.nhs.uk
Tel: 0845 4647
If you have a textphone, you can call the NHS Direct textphone service on 0845 606 46 47

Royal College of General Practitioners

www.rcgp.org.uk

Royal College of Paediatrics and Child Health

www.rcpch.ac.uk

Swine flu information

England: www.nhs.uk or www.direct.gov.uk/swineflu or call the swine flu information line on 0800 1513513. A textphone service is available on 0800 1 513 200 (for people with hearing or speech impairments).
Scotland: www.nhs24.com
Wales: www.nhsdirect.wales.nhs.uk or www.wales.gov.uk/health
Northern Ireland: www.dhsspsni.gov.uk or www.publichealth.hscni.net or call the Northern Ireland Swine Flu Help Line on 0800 0514142.
International: World Health Organization www.who.int/csr/resources/publications/swineflu/en

Index